TREATING HEALTH CARE
How the Canadian System Works and How It Could Work Better

We keep hearing that we need to fix health care. But the prescriptions vary, and to propose helpful changes to health policy requires an understanding of a broad range of issues and interconnected factors. *Treating Health Care* unpacks the key concepts to provide informed discussions that help us understand and diagnose Canada's health care system and to clarify which proposed changes are likely to improve it – and which are not.

This book provides information on topics including determinants of health; how health systems are organized and financed (including international comparisons); health economics; health ethics; and the roles and responsibilities of different stakeholders, including government, providers, and patients. It then addresses some key issues, including equity, efficiency, access and wait times, quality improvement and patient safety, and coverage and payment models. Using analysis rather than advocacy, Raisa B. Deber provides a toolkit to help understand health care and health policy in Canada and place it in an international context.

(UTP Insights)

RAISA B. DEBER is a professor at the Institute of Health Policy, Management and Evaluation at the University of Toronto.

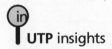
UTP insights

UTP Insights is an innovative collection of brief books offering accessible introductions to the ideas that shape our world. Each volume in the series focuses on a contemporary issue, offering a fresh perspective anchored in scholarship. Spanning a broad range of disciplines in the social sciences and humanities, the books in the UTP Insights series contribute to public discourse and debate and provide a valuable resource for instructors and students.

BOOKS IN THE SERIES

- Raisa B. Deber, *Treating Health Care: How the Canadian System Works and How It Could Work Better*
- Jim Freedman, *A Conviction in Question: The First Trial at the International Criminal Court*
- Christina D. Rosan and Hamil Pearsall, *Growing a Sustainable City? The Question of Urban Agriculture*
- John Joe Schlichtman, Jason Patch, and Marc Lamont Hill, *Gentrifier*
- Robert Chernomas and Ian Hudson, *Economics in the Twenty-First Century: A Critical Perspective*
- Stephen M. Saideman, *Adapting in the Dust: Lessons Learned from Canada's War in Afghanistan*
- Michael R. Marrus, *Lessons of the Holocaust*
- Roland Paris and Taylor Owen (eds.), *The World Won't Wait: Why Canada Needs to Rethink Its International Policies*
- Bessma Momani, *Arab Dawn: Arab Youth and the Demographic Dividend They Will Bring*
- William Watson, *The Inequality Trap: Fighting Capitalism Instead of Poverty*
- Phil Ryan, *After the New Atheist Debate*
- Paul Evans, *Engaging China: Myth, Aspiration, and Strategy in Canadian Policy from Trudeau to Harper*

RAISA B. DEBER

TREATING HEALTH CARE

How the Canadian System Works and How It Could Work Better

UNIVERSITY OF TORONTO PRESS
Toronto Buffalo London

ISBN 978-1-4875-0154-9 (cloth)   ISBN 978-1-4875-2149-3 (paper)

Printed on acid-free, 100% post-consumer recycled paper with vegetable-based inks.

Library and Archives Canada Cataloguing in Publication

Deber, Raisa B., 1949–, author
Treating health care : how the system works and how it could work better /
Raisa B. Deber.

(UTP insights)
Includes bibliographical references and index.
ISBN 978-1-4875-0154-9 (hardcover).   ISBN 978-1-4875-2149-3 (softcover)

1. Medical care – Canada.   2. Medical policy – Canada.   3. Health care
reform – Canada.   I. Title.   II. Series: UTP insights

RA395.C3D375 2017   362.10971   C2017-905073-7

Chapter and title page image: sandr2002/istockphoto

University of Toronto Press acknowledges the financial assistance to its
publishing program of the Canada Council for the Arts and the Ontario Arts
Council, an agency of the Government of Ontario.

Canada Council   Conseil des Arts
for the Arts   du Canada

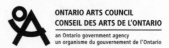

ONTARIO ARTS COUNCIL
CONSEIL DES ARTS DE L'ONTARIO
an Ontario government agency
un organisme du gouvernement de l'Ontario

Funded by the   Financé par le
Government   gouvernement
of Canada   du Canada   Canadä

Contents

Acknowledgments

Health care is a complex but fascinating topic. Over the years, I have been fortunate to have worked on a number of projects, with superb collaborators, that have taught me a lot. I would like to thank the many colleagues and students I have worked with, and learned from, over the years, and my assistant, Kanecy Onate.

I would like to thank University of Toronto Press and Stephen Shapiro for asking me to write this book and for his valuable suggestions, and Dawn Hunter for her excellent copyediting. I appreciate the extremely helpful comments from my test readers Michael I. Bennett, Lady Bolongaita, Adalsteinn (Steini) Brown, Anthony J. Culyer, Bill Dawson, Charles Deber, Mark Dobrow, Gail Donner, Sabha Eftekhary, Margarita Elloso, Selena Lee, Gregory P. Marchildon, Devidas Menon, Mark Rovere, David Rudoler, Stephen Shapiro, and Vidhi R. Thakkar, and the anonymous reviewers.

Finally, my enduring love and thanks to my family, Charles Deber, Jonathan Deber, and Karen Dawson. I couldn't have done it without you.

List of Abbreviations

3Is	ideas, institutions, and interests
A4R	accountability for reasonableness
ADL	activities of daily living
ALC	alternate level of care
BC	British Columbia
CADTH	Canadian Agency for Drugs and Technology in Health
CCAC	Community Care Access Centre
CEA	cost-effectiveness analysis
CHST	Canada Health and Social Transfer
CHA	*Canada Health Act*
CHT	Canada Health Transfer
CIHI	Canadian Institute for Health Information
CST	Canada Social Transfer
CT	computerized tomography (scan)
EPF	*Federal-Provincial Fiscal Arrangements and Established Programs Financing Act*
ED	emergency department
EHR	electronic health record
EMR	electronic medical record
FFS	fee-for-service
FP	for-profit
GDP	gross domestic product
GP	general practitioner
HHR	health human resources

HIDS	*Hospital Insurance and Diagnostic Services Act*
HiT	Health Systems in Transition
HPFB	Health Products and Food Branch of Health Canada
IADL	instrumental activities of daily living
ICER	incremental cost-effectiveness ratio
LHIN	Local Health Integration Network
LPN	licensed practical nurse (see also RPN)
LTC	long-term care
MOHLTC	(Ontario) Ministry of Health and Long-Term Care
MRI	magnetic resonance imaging
MSA	medical savings accounts
NICE	National Institute for Health and Care Excellence
NFP	not-for-profit
NHS	National Health Service (United Kingdom)
OECD	Organisation for Economic Co-operation and Development
OHIP	Ontario Health Insurance Plan
P3	public-private partnership
PC	primary care
PHC	primary health care
PMPRB	Patented Medicine Prices Review Board
PPP	purchasing power parities
PSW	personal support worker
PYLL	potential years of life lost
QALY	quality-adjusted life year
RN	registered nurse
RPN	registered practical nurse
TTO	time trade-off
WHO	World Health Organization
WTP	willingness-to-pay

TREATING HEALTH CARE

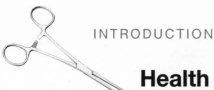

Health Care in Canada: What Works? What Needs to Be Done?

If you ask Canadians for examples of what they are proudest of about their country, universal health care is usually high on the list, along with hockey (although they will usually insist you not call it "ice hockey"), maple syrup, and their being so polite. This pride has led to considerable discomfort when international rankings place Canadian health care in the middle, or even near the bottom, of the pack. We still look very good compared with the United States, but so does everyone else.

Seeing that ranking, in turn, usually leads to cries to fix the system, although one could argue how much these cries have led to meaningful change. Calls for reform focus on a number of issues, but particular attention is usually focused on costs, access, and quality.

This book attempts to clarify some of the concepts and share the background information needed to understand some major issues surrounding health care and evaluate where we might (or might not) want to go. Understanding health policy requires knowledge that spans a broad range of topics. This book aims to fill a gap in the existing literature by providing brief, accurate descriptions of key topics for intelligent readers without assuming that they already know the details. I also try to highlight what factors I think need to be balanced in making wise (or at least not foolish) decisions. Accordingly, this book is not a textbook on health economics or political science, although I do include some references for the interested reader. Neither is it a description of where I think Canada's health system should go, although again I do reference some good examples. This book instead tries to avoid advocacy in favour of analysis. As an experienced teacher of health policy, my philosophy has always been that it is not my job to tell you what you should want, but it is my job to tell you whether a particular approach is likely to take you where you want to go. As such, the book provides a toolkit to help you understand or diagnose Canada's health care system and clarify which proposed treatment options are likely to help (or harm) it. As tools, they should remain helpful for assessing options, even as new issues arise.

Health care policy analysts are fond of acronyms. I have tried to be moderate in my use of them but felt it might be useful to indicate some of the more common terminology. For your convenience, a List of Abbreviations is included after the Table of Contents.

The book also tries to link the concepts discussed to how they might help you understand how to implement some commonly suggested reforms that I do think might be valuable:

- Make people healthier and help them stay healthy.
- Improve how services are coordinated and improve the quality of care, including patient safety.
- Change how we organize our system, including how we pay for care (including who pays for what) and how we deliver it (including doing something about wait lists and access).
- Become more efficient, to get better value for money.

The concepts and information presented here are an effort to encourage us to make things better, without making them worse. The material draws on a number of research projects (including some I was involved with), as well as some key concepts mentioned in my book *Case Studies in Canadian Health Policy and Management*, particularly in the first chapter.[1]

Chapter Outline

Chapter 1 of this book defines some key concepts, including policy and what affects it. It talks about what is meant by health and by health care, and what are called the *determinants of health* (also known as the things that are associated with making us more, or less, healthy). The chapter introduces the concepts of *public goods* and *externalities* as they affect potential government roles and responsibilities. It provides some insight into the first reform suggestion: make people healthier and help them stay healthy.

Chapter 2 looks at health care, including the many silos within which care is delivered, and who delivers it, including what it means to be a *professional*. It briefly discusses health human resources and how to determine how many of various kinds of providers we might need. This chapter provides some background for the second reform suggestion: improve how services are coordinated and improve the quality of care, including patient safety.

Chapter 3 focuses on the third reform suggestion by examining various ways that health care systems can be organized, including how they are paid for (*financing*), how care is delivered (*delivery*), and how providers can be reimbursed (*allocation*). It includes some background on what insurance is and how health care differs from other goods and services. It also clarifies what is meant by *public* and *private*, and how these dimensions come together to describe different types of health care systems.

Chapter 4 turns to Canada and how we have chosen to organize care. It notes how the way Canada has distributed power between the federal and provincial/territorial levels of government affects how we can (and cannot) manage health care. It also gives some material about the current rules affecting what has to be covered, with a focus on the *Canada Health Act*, and concludes with some information on how much it costs and how this varies across members of the population. In particular, I show that averages can be misleading, since health expenditures are highly skewed, with a small number of "high spenders" (also known as sick people) accounting for a high proportion of health costs.

Chapter 5 builds on the description of different models of health care in Chapter 3 to look at how the Canadian system compares internationally. We focus on three examples – the United Kingdom, Germany, and the United States – that use three of the other major approaches to financing and delivering care. Looking at some key indicators, we see where Canada does relatively well and where there is room for improvement.

Chapter 6 looks at the fourth reform suggestion – become more efficient, to get better value for money – examining how we might decide what is worth paying for, including short overviews of health economics and health care ethics. It briefly describes what is meant by cost-effectiveness, how we might translate economic analysis into policy, and the importance of balancing risks and benefits (using screening as an example). It also discusses who should decide and the role of the patient.

Chapter 7 looks at some pressing issues, such as equity, access (including wait times), quality improvement and patient safety, and accountability. It should help with diagnosing what aspects of health care in Canada might require treatment.

Chapter 8 turns to possible treatments; it analyses what the information in this book might mean for some common proposals for health reform, and where we might go from here. Using some of the concepts and information provided, we look at the reforms suggested above. The treatments analysed include making people healthier, improving how we coordinate services and the quality of care, changing how we pay for care (including allowing private payment), changing what we cover, changing how we pay providers and deliver care, and improving efficiency.

Careful examination makes it clear that the devil is usually in the details. In particular, most policy questions are about trade-offs. As such, there is usually not one right answer. However, there are many wrong ones, some of which are examined in the subsequent chapters. In particular, I suggest that attention to such proposals as making people healthier, improving how services are coordinated (which is usually called *service integration*), improving quality of care and patient safety, and modifying what is covered are likely to be helpful, whereas encouraging more private payment is likely to make things worse. My analysis also suggests that the sky is not falling, although there are certainly many things we could – and hopefully will – do to make Canadian health care even healthier.

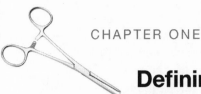

CHAPTER ONE

Defining Our Terms: What Is Health Policy? What Is Health?

Policy and What Affects It

To talk about policy, it is helpful to first define what is meant by the term. *Policy* has multiple definitions, but they basically boil down to describing what we want to accomplish. One way to define policy is as "a set of interrelated decisions taken by a political actor or group of actors concerning the selection of goals and the means of achieving them within a specified situation where these decisions should, in principle, be within the power of these actors to achieve."[1] This means that policies are not always written down (unlike, for example, a policy and procedure manual in a workplace). The selected policy could involve deciding not to change anything, which is sometimes termed *non-decisions*.[2] Because we are talking about intentions rather than results, policies do not necessarily achieve the desired goals. Policy issues also vary in their complexity. As noted US political scientist Aaron Wildavsky observed, when dealing with difficult policy decisions, we rarely solve them.[3] Instead, we often replace one set of problems with a new set of problems; under those circumstances, success means preferring the new problems to the old ones.

One way to analyse how policy is developed is to focus on what policy analysts often call the 3Is – ideas, institutions, and interests.

Ideas deal with values and with what we want to do. Ideas accordingly help structure how we see the world and what we think is important.

Institutions are the structures within which decisions will be made, including who will and will not be at the table, and the rules of the game. For example, decisions affecting health can be made at many levels, including by governments passing laws and regulations, civil servants interpreting these policies, courts ruling on legal disputes, and individuals and providers (which may include hospitals and doctors) deciding on care plans. The participants and rules of the game can vary considerably depending on where those decisions are made.

Interests refers to the stakeholders – those who can affect or be affected by what that organization does or what policy is adopted. Political scientists distinguish between what are sometimes called *concentrated interests*, those who have a major stake in a particular issue, and *diffuse interests*, those for whom that issue is just one of many possible things they might be involved in. Not surprisingly, concentrated interests are far more likely to participate in trying to influence policy in their areas of concern. The distinction between facts and values is important to keep in mind; people are not entitled to their own facts but may indeed differ in what outcomes they would prefer. In addition, because different interests often stress different ideas, changes in institutions may, in turn, strongly influence who is involved in making policy decisions and hence which ideas are most likely to win. In this volume, we will try to cast some light on these concepts when they are useful to help understand how health care might be treated.

One thing to keep in mind when analysing health policy is the need to specify what we are trying to accomplish, recognizing that, as already noted, we are usually talking about trade-offs. Usually, we want more than one thing. Political scientist Deborah Stone has suggested four key policy objectives, which she notes are not always compatible.[4] The first, which she terms "security," is satisfying our minimum human needs; this may include such things as having a place to live, enough nutritious food to eat, and protection against bombs falling from the sky. The second, which she terms "liberty," is to allow people to do what they want, as long as they do not harm others. This can quickly clash with the goal of security, particularly if people need help from others to meet their basic needs. One common example is the extent to which the better off should be taxed to help pay for such things as social housing for the poor (or the healthy should be taxed to pay for health care for the sick). The third goal, which Stone terms "equity," is defined as "treating likes alike" and can rapidly turn into arguments about what counts as likes. Finally, what she calls "efficiency" is getting the most for the money spent. Unlike the previous three objectives, efficiency can be seen as a second-order goal, since it only comes into play after you decide that you want that particular output. As we will see in Chapter 6, economic analysis primarily concerns itself with efficiency.

It is important to recognize the distinction between policy advocacy and policy analysis. People often differ in the priority they assign to various policy goals. Good policy analysts do not assume that their goals should be given the highest priority but can help clarify how likely it is that a specific policy approach would achieve particular goals. Policy advocates, in contrast, begin with the assumption that the goals they prefer are the ones that should be adopted and marshal (often selective) evidence to support them. This book focuses on policy analysis.

Another set of key concepts deals with how we can achieve those desired outcomes. What policy analysts refer to as *policy instruments* are the tools available to help achieve the selected policy goals. These tools can be classified in a number of ways, which attach different terms to similar concepts. We will use the typology suggested by Canadian political scientists Bruce Doern and Richard Phidd, which classifies these tools in terms of how much coercion they involve.[5] To illustrate, we will apply these instruments to the policy problem of doing something about obesity, which can be harmful to people's health.

The least coercive policy instrument is to do nothing. We might argue that people should be free to eat whatever they would like and decide not to do anything about obesity. Next, we might choose to use some of the tools in what Doern and Phidd call the "exhortation" category, which would encourage people to behave in a certain way without forcing them to do so. Examples might include developing public education programs to persuade people to eat healthy foods and to exercise, or using symbolic gestures, such as highlighting political leaders shaking hands with student athletes. The "expenditure" tools involve spending money; for example, we could subsidize healthy school lunches. The "taxation" tools involve using tax policy to encourage or discourage certain activities; for example, people could get tax deductions for enrolling their children in physical activity programs. Government could also impose taxes on foods it thinks are unhealthy (such as sugary soft drinks). The "regulation" tools involve setting rules that will encourage or penalize particular activities. For example, manufacturers could be compelled to publish lists of ingredients on their food packaging that would allow people to make more informed choices. Governments could also ban certain types of foods deemed to be unhealthy (as some jurisdictions did with trans-fats). Finally, the "public ownership" tools involve government taking over an activity and directly running it; one example might be opening a public skating rink to encourage people to exercise.

Most health care systems make heavy use of all these policy instruments, depending on the policy goals and the institutions in charge of the policy initiatives, recognizing that different institutions will have access to different policy instruments. For example, regulation is relied on to control who provides care and to ensure it is of sufficiently high quality, but the ability to employ this instrument depends on having the ability to enforce these regulations. Taxation may allow some personal expenditures for purchasing supplementary health care services (or private insurance) to be tax deductible. Expenditure is used to pay for many services, including physician and hospital services. Exhortation is used to try to help people live healthier lives. Public ownership can be used to operate some services, particularly if there is good reason to believe that the private sector is unwilling (or unable) to do this in a satisfactory manner.

Health Care and Health

In its simplest form, *health care* can be defined as services aimed at improving (or maintaining) health, which may also include preventing disease. Defining what *health* is, however, is not that simple. One common definition from the World Health Organization (WHO) defined health as "a state of complete physical, mental and social well-being and not merely the absence of disease or infirmity."[6] Using that definition, everything can be seen as health. Are you happily married? Do you like your job? Did your favourite hockey team win a big game? If the answers relate to your complete physical, mental, and social well-being, by that definition, we're talking about health. At the other extreme, some define health primarily in terms of delivering sickness care. Usually, when we talk about a health care system, we are referring to sickness care.

Public Health and Determinants of Health: Keeping Us Healthy

Canada has been among the world leaders in recognizing the importance of multiple factors in promoting health. Back in 1974, the Lalonde Report[7] argued that the health of populations was affected by the following four categories of factors (which it termed "fields"): human biology, environment, lifestyle, and health care organization. *Human biology* referred to the biological causes of disease, including genetic inheritance. *Environment* referred to both physical and social environmental factors over which individuals would have little or no control, including such things as air and water quality. *Lifestyle* referred to personal decisions that could contribute to how healthy a person was, including whether the person smoked, drank too much alcohol, abused other substances, ate healthy food, and got enough exercise. Health care organization referred to clinical services to patients.

Subsequent reports have further subdivided these categories into multiple factors that contribute to what soon came to be known as the *determinants of health*. There are multiple lists with similar items, although the precise labels given to each factor can vary somewhat. For example, the Public Health Agency of Canada lists the following 12 "key determinants of health": income and social status; social support networks; education and literacy; employment/working conditions; social environments; physical environments; personal health practices and coping skills; healthy child development; biology and genetic endowment; health services; gender; and culture.[8] All these factors but biology and health services are often called the "social determinants of health."[9] The WHO has a similar list.[10]

Determinants of health include an extensive set of factors. Dealing with them would involve almost everyone – not only all branches of government but basically everyone we interact with.

Within health care, much of the responsibility for dealing with the determinants of health lies with what is usually called *public health*. One commonly used definition of public health talks about the importance of "the maintenance and improvement of the health of all the people."[11] Indeed, an influential 1986 document reflecting efforts by the WHO to achieve "health for all" is known as the Ottawa Charter.[12] A similar concept is termed *population health*, which also stresses the importance of seeking to improve the health of the entire population by acting on "the broad range of factors and conditions that have a strong influence on our health."[13] Under this definition, almost everything would qualify as population health. As one of many examples of the complexities arising from trying to improve population health, the Canadian Senate struck a Subcommittee on Population Health, chaired by Senator Keon. The final report, issued in June 2009, focused heavily on reporting and evaluation, and recommended that the prime minister should establish a committee on population health. Its report explicitly argued that this committee should be chaired by the prime minister, and should "comprise the relevant departmental ministers including, but not limited to: Human Resources and Skills Development, Indian and Northern Affairs, Finance, Health, Environment, Justice, Agriculture and Agri-Food, Industry, Public Health Agency, and Status of Women."[14] (As of this writing, the report has still not been acted on.)

A related activity often falling within the public health definition includes making sure that someone collects and analyses data to allow us to monitor health and disease. This analysis allows us to understand how healthy we are (or are not), what problems we might need to deal with (including surveillance activities to allow us to detect new outbreaks of disease before they spread too widely), and the extent to which these data vary across jurisdictions. Note that the data can be – and are – collected by and used by a multitude of organizations, not just those labelled as public health. Coordinating the data is not simple. It requires multiple bodies to agree on how they will report things, to whom, and who will pay for it. Often, this is easier wished for than done.

In practice, those dealing with health care tend to use narrower definitions of public health that focus on preventing diseases. Disease prevention is often divided into three categories. *Primary prevention* tries to stop disease or injury before it happens; examples include not only encouraging healthy eating and physical activity but also banning the use of hazardous activities or products. *Secondary prevention* tries to reduce the impact of an existing disease or injury (e.g., through early detection and treatment), whereas *tertiary prevention* tries to help people manage long-term health problems and thus improve their quality of life. Public health organizations tend to focus on primary prevention. In addition to the multiple benefits of keeping people healthier, this approach can also be extremely cost-effective. One ongoing problem with selling a focus on primary prevention, however, is that success is often invisible, since we are rarely aware of the disasters that didn't happen. This can sometimes lead to complacency and even erode success. One example is immunization; people who have not seen friends paralysed by polio may not see why they (or their children) should receive their polio vaccinations until an outbreak which should have been preventable occurs. Another is water treatment, in which governments may neglect maintaining infrastructure because citizens prefer not to pay higher taxes, until their children begin suffering the effects of lead poisoning. Calls to reduce regulation – such as those advocated by the Trump administration in the United States – focus on the desirability of reducing the burden on business but may lead to "penny wise pound foolish" decisions that ignore long-term effects of failing to prevent such problems.

In many jurisdictions, the activities carried out by the organizations known as public health often go beyond this focus on prevention. As one example, public health agencies may be heavily involved in the provision of services to target populations, usually for populations or services not covered by health insurance systems. In the United States, this means that public health is often responsible for the care of indigent populations. In Canada, in addition to the health protection and promotion activities noted above, public health in many jurisdictions is often involved in filling service gaps; depending on the jurisdiction, this can include such activities as providing services to vulnerable newborn children and their parents, sexual health education and family planning, and preventive and clinical dental health services to vulnerable populations. Indeed, in some jurisdictions, public health may even become involved in providing healthy lunches to schoolchildren.

At the policy level, a broad focus on the determinants of health can point to various ways to best improve population health. One possible set of interventions could focus on improving the environment (e.g., curbing air pollution, making cities more walkable, or wiping out mosquitos that might spread infectious diseases). The field of health promotion focuses on lifestyle and how best to help individuals improve their health by encouraging healthy eating, exercise, and not smoking, and providing people with social support. Accordingly, the policy levers to try to improve the health of a population will often extend beyond the health care system. For example, improved design of cars (including mandating use of seat belts) and more careful attention to road design has greatly reduced motor vehicle deaths in many countries, including Canada. Implementing and enforcing building codes can reduce the risks from fires, collapsing balconies, or exposure to toxins, such as asbestos. Regulating food safety can reduce health problems from contaminated products. Encouraging people not to smoke or abuse substances is likely to make them healthier. Attention to public safety and building a strong and nurturing community can minimize crime rates and decrease the risk of people being shot or bombed. Clearly, deciding on the extent to which public action is justified can be controversial. For example, ensuring that people have adequate housing and good food is clearly critical to their health, but this has rarely translated into acceptance that everyone should be entitled to have enough money to live on, regardless of whether or not they are working.

The health care system per se rarely deals with most of the determinants of health, although they are extremely important. Instead, it focuses primarily (although not exclusively) on health care services, often called sickness care, whose scope will be defined in Chapter 2.

Roles and Responsibilities: What Should Government Do?

An ongoing policy debate concerns the limits of government. When should it become involved, and when should it leave people alone? This clearly relates to ideas about how to balance different policy objectives. Someone who stresses individual liberty, for example, will be reluctant to pay taxes to benefit others, whereas those placing more value on equity and security may see helping others as a good use of their money. However, one clear justification for government involvement that almost everyone accepts relates to the concept known as *public goods*.

The term public goods (also referred to as *collective goods*) is commonly used in the policy analysis and economics literature; it is not the same as being good for the public. Public goods (and their opposite, private goods) are defined in terms of two inherent characteristics: *rivalry in consumption* and *excludability in ownership and use*.

Rivalry in consumption means that what one person consumes cannot be consumed by anyone else. *Excludability* means that some particular person has exclusive control over that item. For example, my sunglasses are a private good because when I wear them, no one else can (rivalry in consumption) and, because I own them, I determine who gets to wear them at any particular time (excludability). Public goods are accordingly defined as being non-rivalrous or non-excludable (although pure public goods are both). If one person breathes clean air, that does not prevent others from doing so; clean air thus meets the non-rivalrous criterion for being a public good (although to be precise, you cannot breathe the same molecules that are in my lungs). In contrast, clean water may indeed be rivalrous; water can be packaged, and what one person drinks cannot be consumed by another. Similarly, a non-excludable good cannot be restricted to only those who want to (or can) pay for it. If it is there, anyone can use it. National defence is a clear example of non-excludability; everyone, not only those willing to pay, will be protected from foreign invasion. A more debatable example is public roads. In practice, these are usually non-excludable, since after a road is built, people can go ahead and use it whether they have paid for it directly or not. However, a road can be made private by limiting its use to those who pay for it (e.g., a toll highway). One side effect of the growth of the Internet was that books and music were harder to keep rivalrous or excludable. If I had a vinyl record album and you borrowed it, I would no longer have it. However, once music became electronic, I could give you a copy and still have one myself. The same applies to electronic books. Those who sell books and music tried – with fairly minimal success – to limit such sharing, but technology has basically turned these products into public goods, to the financial detriment of those trying to earn a living by providing them. (One option that musicians still have is to spend a great deal of time on the road giving concerts, since concert tickets are still both rivalrous and excludable.)

One key aspect of public health that, as we will see, clearly falls into the category of public goods relates to preventing and managing communicable diseases. Communicable diseases are transmitted through direct or indirect contact with an infected individual; they are caused by microorganisms, including bacteria, viruses, parasites, and fungi. Such pathogens can cause infections in various organs of the human body, which can cause complications arising from the infection itself or from the host's immunological response to the infectious organism or both. Historically, infections have been one of the major causes of death. However, in the twentieth century, a series of innovations, including the use of water sanitation, better hygiene, vaccination, and anti-microbial drugs, resulted in a global reduction of infectious illness (although the rates are still far too high in many developing countries). In most developed countries, this reduction was large enough that the major causes of death became chronic diseases, such as cancer and cardiovascular illness. Indeed, for a while there was a premature belief that the era of infectious diseases was over. However, infectious disease has made a comeback over the last 50 years, including new infections, such as Zika virus, Ebola, SARS (severe acute respiratory syndrome), West Nile virus, and human immuno-deficiency virus (HIV), as well as a resurgence of older infections, such as tuberculosis and measles. An individual's decision about whether to purchase an immunization is not a public good, since it is rivalrous; if I get the vaccine, no one else can have that dose.

In contrast, control of infectious diseases at the community level meets the definition of a public good because of what is called *herd immunity*: once a high enough proportion of the population is im-mune to a communicable disease, the infectious agent finds it harder to find a new host to infect. Accordingly, the disease becomes much less likely to be transmitted. In turn, this reduces the risk to the rest of the population who are not yet immune, since they are less likely to come into contact with people who might infect them. Herd immunity is particularly advantageous for people who have impaired immunity and cannot be immunized safely for certain conditions (e.g., children being treated for cancer usually should not receive some vaccines). One ongoing policy dilemma is referred to as the *free rider problem*; purely rational individuals, when this term is defined as people acting only in their own narrow self-interest, have an incentive to avoid pay-ing for public goods, knowing that they will still be able to obtain the benefits as long as others agree to pay. For example, rational individu-als would selfishly decline immunization, avoiding the personal costs and the potential risks of side effects, as long as enough of their neighbours were immunized to allow them to still capture the bene-fits through herd immunity. However, if enough people behave this way, herd immunity will disappear, placing everyone at risk again.

A related concept is called *externalities*. Externalities occur when private costs and benefits are not the same as social costs and bene-fits. Some of these externalities can be positive (e.g., herd immunity protects everyone in a community, whether they were immunized or not). Some externalities can be negative (e.g., pollution or global warming allows the polluters to transfer their costs and harms to oth-ers). A key policy issue is that, without some mechanism to address externalities, there may be a tendency to under-invest in public goods with positive externalities and to allow people to impose negative externalities on others. That is why even advocates of minimal government will usually – but not always – accept government involvement in addressing public goods (e.g., national defence, protection against communicable diseases, prohibition against dumping polluting material into public waterways), both to deal with externalities and to prevent free riders. However, Institutions are key. One ongoing problem is that there are few mechanisms to enforce regulations across political boundaries. Someone polluting the air or water in one jurisdiction can impose massive externalities on their neighbours in other jurisdictions, but unless these jurisdictions cooperate, there may be no way to stop this from happening. This has been a major barrier to dealing with environmental issues, including climate change and, to a lesser extent, water pollution, since one bad apple can indeed spoil multiple bunches.

It is important to recognize that, under this definition, many things that are good for the public would not qualify as public goods. For example, although having universal health care services financed by governments is sometimes referred to as a public good, it does not meet the definition, since most health care services delivered to individuals fit the definition of private goods. If I break my arm, any care I receive would be both rivalrous and excludable. The category of *merit goods* or *club goods* is sometimes applied to goods and services, such as health care, that do not meet the definition of public goods but are still considered good for the public. One rationale for calling something a merit good occurs when people are uncomfortable allowing others to suffer. However, there are often differences in who is seen as qualifying for help. As one example, even people who want to help may want to limit this to recipients who satisfy certain conditions (e.g., being citizens of the same country, or being a close friend or family member). However, as the often acrimonious debates over social policy make clear, support for such expenditures is by no means universal. In contrast, it is usually easier to gain public consensus if a policy goal is clearly a public good (or can be portrayed as one). As noted above, controlling communicable diseases is clearly a public good. Although health care services, such as access to hospital care, do not really fit the definition of public goods, advocates for ensuring universal coverage may argue that since having a well-functioning health care system to prevent, identify, and treat these diseases is also essential, we should treat it as though it were a public good.

Similar arguments can be made for anti-poverty strategies. Arguably, eliminating homelessness and ensuring that everyone has enough healthy food to eat is a good thing to do for its own sake. This can be extended to suggest that such programs are cost-effective; desperate people may become criminals, and the costs of imprisoning people would probably be higher than the costs of giving them the resources needed to allow them to become productive members of society. (Similar arguments have successfully been made for making public schools free.) How convincing these arguments are will therefore affect whether people see paying for services for others as also being in their own self-interest.

We will return to how policies can help make people healthier in Chapter 8. First, however, we need to examine the components of health care and the different ways we can choose to pay for it, especially health insurance.

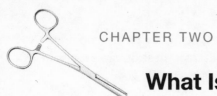

CHAPTER TWO

What Is Health Care?

As noted health economist Robert Evans wrote, we do not want to buy health care; we want to buy health.[1] One problem is that we do not know what economists call the *production function*, which connects the inputs (the resources needed to provide health care) to the outputs (health).[2] Several categories of services constitute what we often refer to as health care. Too often, these exist in separate silos with minimal coordination, as well as different rules about who will pay for what.

Types of Services (The Silos)

Sickness care is not homogeneous. One way to classify it is to focus on the level of care, which is often described as primary, secondary, or tertiary (or quaternary). The terms *primary health care* (or PHC) and *primary care* (or PC) are commonly used to designate the initial point of entry into a health care system. Primary health care includes not only primary care clinical services but also health promotion, disease prevention, and rehabilitation. More commonly, we speak of primary care, which has a less expansive definition, focusing on the provision of services to diagnose, treat, and manage diseases. Primary care services are usually (although not exclusively) performed by general practitioners (GPs, who may also be called family doctors or family physicians). Primary care services usually include check-ups, certain preventive services (including immunizations in some jurisdictions), and ongoing treatment of common ailments. Increasingly, primary care is delivered by interdisciplinary teams, where doctors work with various combinations of nurses (possibly including nurse practitioners), physician assistants, social workers, dieticians, or other professionals. Depending on the population being served, primary care can also be delivered by larger organizations (with a variety of names, including community health centres), which also try to deal with some of the broader determinants of health. For example, such organizations may also liaise with other community organizations to link with community housing, services for immigrants, or mental health services.

Primary care has been shown to be a critical part of high-performing health care.[3] Ideally, every person will be affiliated with a primary care provider. This affiliation implies that the designated providers will provide comprehensive services to their patients whenever these services are needed, will help ensure that care is coordinated, and will refer patients to specialized care when it is needed. Primary care thus frequently operates as a gatekeeper to other health care services. In practice, patients who are not sufficiently affiliated with a primary care provider can use walk-in clinics, where there may not be much continuity in terms of who provides the services, or may decide to go to hospital emergency rooms. In an effort to encourage continuity of care, newer models of primary care are being employed in many countries (and in many Canadian provinces) that require patients to formally register with a provider (which could be a particular physician or a primary care organization); this is usually called *patient rostering*. In some other models, the rostering may be more informal; for example, the payer might look at the billing records to see where a patient normally goes to receive care, and consider patients to be *virtually rostered* to whatever provider they usually see. Rostering is seen as a key mechanism for making sure that each patient is linked with primary care providers who can help coordinate their care.

The next level of care refers to more specialized services, which can be offered in multiple settings. For example, if primary care providers suspect people have vision problems, they may refer them to an ophthalmologist. If someone needs surgery, they will usually be referred to a surgeon. Some specialized services may be offered in an office setting, while others may require the supports available in a hospital. (*Ambulatory care* is sometimes used to refer to all services given outside of hospitals, which would include both primary care and those specialized services that are offered on an outpatient basis.)

Hospitals provide even more specialized care. Depending on how specialized the hospital is, such care can be described as secondary, tertiary, or quaternary care. Secondary services are available in any hospital. In contrast, tertiary care is more complex and requires specialized expertise that is not always available in all hospitals. Such care is often referred to as subspecialty services. Examples include cancer treatment, cardiac surgery, or treatment for severe burns. The line between tertiary and quaternary care is blurry and depends on how specialized a particular service is; quaternary care may include gathering information about new therapies (usually through clinical trials) to see whether they are sufficiently safe and effective for more widespread use. Many tertiary/quaternary hospitals are also teaching hospitals and thus are involved in training the next generation of clinicians. Depending on how the health care system operates in a particular jurisdiction, people usually need to be referred (typically by a physician) to receive such specialized services, as opposed to being able to refer themselves to primary care. However, people usually have the option of referring themselves to an emergency room or urgent care centre and allowing the doctors there to refer them to specialized care, if appropriate.

A related category is emergency services, which deals with situations that are potentially life-threatening. (*Urgent care* is often used to refer to problems that are less severe but cannot wait for an appointment with a family doctor. Examples might include severe headaches or severe back pain.) Ambulance services deal with emergencies and if necessary can transport people to the most suitable location to treat them. Ambulances may deal directly with emergencies in the community and then drive people to a suitable hospital; their skilled staff (including paramedics and emergency medical technicians) may be able to begin treatment en route. Ambulances may also be used to transport people between hospitals if the initial hospital does not have the specialized expertise needed to treat that patient.

Long-term care (LTC) refers to a set of health, personal care, and social services; however, unlike acute care, which is required for a relatively short time, LTC services are often (but not always) required on a sustained basis. LTC is sometimes divided into three categories: *acute care substitution* allows people to be discharged from acute hospitals to the community and still receive the services they need; *long-term care substitution* serves those who might otherwise have to be in LTC institutions; and *prevention/maintenance* keeps people healthy enough to remain out of institutions.[4] Accordingly, LTC may be delivered within a specialized facility (e.g., nursing home, home for the aged) or in the community (e.g., in-home services, community support services, supportive housing). LTC services may thus exist in two silos – one for LTC institutions and another for home and community care. We will use LTC in this book to refer to both of these settings. LTC may include help with some clinical services, including wound care or administration of medications, but goes beyond sickness care to include other elements of the determinants of health. By definition, it includes food and shelter. What are often called *social supports* include help with things like doing the shopping, the laundry, and cleaning. What are sometimes called activities of daily living (ADL) involve the sorts of tasks that people normally do but may need help with, including things like functional mobility (e.g., the ability to walk, get in and out of bed) and personal care (e.g., helping people take a bath, get dressed, or eat). Instrumental activities of daily living (IADL) also help people live independently and may involve help with shopping, housework, transportation, or meal preparation. Such activities evoke the circle of life – just as all children need and should receive such personal support services, as we age, we may again need help. Another key need is companionship. Although some of these community-based LTC services are provided by paid workers, most of it is done by informal caregivers, which may include family members, friends, or volunteers. The community-based LTC category may thus include various forms of support for these valuable but unpaid workers. From a practical point of view, depending on the jurisdiction, many of the services and activities in the community-based LTC category may be the responsibility of different government departments or agencies, which may present problems in coordinating policy. As will be noted in the following chapters, there are also major practical and ethical questions about who should pay for which components of LTC. These decisions usually depend heavily on the ideas portion of the 3Is, that is, on our values about what are public and private responsibilities.

Other silos refer to types of care rather than to where they are delivered. These are partly defined in terms of the specialties involved and partly in terms of the body parts being treated. For example, rehabilitation refers to treatments designed to facilitate recovery, including physical therapy, occupational therapy, and speech-language therapy. Rehabilitation can be delivered in inpatient, outpatient, or LTC settings (including the home). Similarly, pharmaceuticals are an important element in preventing, treating, and managing disease, and account for a considerable proportion of health expenditures. Other types of services include diagnostic imaging, dental care, mental health care, palliative care, complementary and alternative medicine, vision care, and so on.

One ongoing question is how these various services are organized and how they work together. Policymakers often speak of *integration* and *coordination* (and sometimes use such terms as *continuity of care*). Although these terms can be defined in myriad ways, one key element refers to how well the different providers work together, as well as on how (and by whom) they are paid. From the patients' point of view, a central question is whether the providers share information so that the patient does not have to keep answering the same questions over and over again. Payers and managers may want to focus on such questions as how the care is organized, whether the services are provided at the same location, and whether they fall under the same management structure. *Integration* usually refers to whether multiple organizations have been brought together into one management structure, since certain things will be far simpler if the providers are all within a single organization. Distinction can also be made between *horizontal integration* among team members at the same level of care (or among organizations providing a similar level of care affiliated under one management structure) and *vertical integration* across different levels of care (e.g., linking primary, secondary, and tertiary care).[5] Clearly, the policy issues will vary. Conversely, *coordination* relates to whether multiple groups can cooperate with one another. As will be discussed in subsequent chapters, the ability to coordinate often depends on the extent to which we employ a competitive market.

Who Provides Health Care? Defining Professions

Health care can be delivered by a vast array of providers. These providers often vary in the sorts of training they have, the tasks they perform, and where they work.

One useful concept in examining those providers is that of a *profession*. Although there is a considerable body of literature that tries to define what makes something a profession,[6] most agree that professions are characterized by the following elements. The work relies on a systematic body of knowledge that must be learned and is almost always taught in recognized educational institutions. There must be a mechanism for testing and assessing whether this knowledge has been mastered, recognizing that much of this knowledge might be sufficiently esoteric that only someone else with the same training is able to properly judge whether the candidate has indeed mastered it. The services provided by these professionals to members of the public can place their recipients at risk of harm if they are not done properly. However, unlike other consumer transactions, the customer is not in a position to judge whether the person performing that service is doing it properly (or sometimes even if the service is necessary); this is sometimes described as an *agency relationship* between the client and the provider. As one example, if I hire you to build a bridge and you build it badly, it may collapse and place those using that bridge at risk. However, if I am not a trained engineer, I am not likely to know whether you are building it properly until it collapses. An additional complexity is that, particularly in health care, outcomes alone are often not sufficient to monitor performance, because people can have bad outcomes even if the care was excellent and, conversely, can get better even when receiving poor quality care. One example is an early attempt to rate hospitals performing cardiac surgery where the hospitals with the best reputations initially appeared to have much worse results; closer examination revealed that this was because they were treating much sicker patients.

One way of handling this asymmetry of information between those who provide care and those who receive it is to develop a professional body that issues certification to its members and oversees their activities. This means that amateurs cannot apply; to work in that profession, you must become a member of the professional body. In health care, these bodies are often called colleges, and the professions are known as *regulated health professions*. Because you need to have that knowledge to judge performance, these bodies are self-regulating (meaning that they are largely although often not entirely made up of people who hold that professional qualification). However, as noted in our earlier discussion of institutions, these regulatory bodies do not have the ability to enforce these rules unless government has given them the authority to do so. This means that the relevant level of government must pass legislation that grants specified powers to these professional bodies. Frequently, colleges are also given responsibility for overseeing the professional practices of their members, including handling complaints when these occur. Because the distinction between a profession and a skilled occupation is not always clear, which professions are recognized, and what they can or cannot do, often varies by jurisdiction. Considerable variation exists across jurisdictions in how these professions are regulated, including who is in charge and the extent to which members of the profession can control the process or are monitored by regulators who are not members of their profession. These procedures are one key element in trying to deal with the improve quality of care element of our second reform suggestion.

There are several dimensions to designating something as a profession. The simplest is what is called *protection of title*. For example, in Ontario, you cannot refer to yourself as a physiotherapist unless you are a member of the College of Physiotherapists of Ontario. This is similar, but not identical, to the ability of religious organizations to control who is authorized to call themselves a priest/minister/rabbi/imam of that denomination, since in most jurisdictions government would not enforce any sanctions these bodies might impose against people who violate their rules. As an example of an occupation that does not have protection of title, in most jurisdictions, you can call yourself a housepainter without formal training or certification. A more complex dimension relates to who is allowed to do particular things; the rationale for controlling certain acts is that the public will be placed at risk unless that act is performed by someone who has been certified as capable of doing it. For health care, Ontario refers to these as "controlled acts" and has passed legislation that specifies that certain controlled acts can only be carried out by members of particular professions. For example, you are not allowed to perform surgery unless you are a physician and your professional college also agrees that you have the necessary skills. Similar restrictions are placed on who can prescribe medications that are designated as prescription drugs. However, many of the activities performed by regulated professionals may not be controlled acts. For example, you do not need to be a speech-language pathologist to try to help someone speak more clearly (although you may not be as effective as someone with the appropriate training). Similarly, hairdressers, bartenders, and friends can try to help people cope with difficult circumstances without being registered psychologists.

Professionalism can be a contentious concept. Opponents of giving professional designation often note that restricting who can enter a profession is a form of elitism; those on the inside usually can make more money and enjoy higher social status. Supporters of professionalism stress the importance of competence and trust. Deciding what should be considered a profession accordingly can be contentious, and, as noted above, what qualifies varies across jurisdictions. In general, certain professions (e.g., medicine, nursing, law, engineering) are classified as professions and registered in almost all jurisdictions, while others may not be.

One issue is whether these groups can still call themselves professions in jurisdictions that do not recognize their regulatory body. Naturopathy is one example; it is regulated in some Canadian provinces and US states, but not in others. Similarly, people who want to call themselves naturopathic physicians can take a variety of training programs, some (but not all) of which have been accredited by their accrediting body. If they graduate from one of those programs, they can take provincial or state board examinations and register with that regulatory body. The website for the Canadian Association of Naturopathic Doctors warns that people who have completed correspondence programs, which are not accredited, are not eligible to take these examinations, but those people may indeed practise in many jurisdictions, although they usually are not allowed to perform controlled acts (including writing prescriptions).[7]

Other work can be referred to as *expert occupations* (or *skilled trades*); these may or may not be designated as professions, depending on the jurisdiction. Examples include computer programmers, firefighters, teachers, and real estate agents. Variation may also exist in whether volunteers who may not be formally trained or certified are allowed to perform particular tasks. In Ontario, for example, electrical work must be done by certified electricians, whereas carpentry (at the time of writing) does not have to be done by certified carpenters.

Much health care is delivered by people who are not classified as health professionals. One example is LTC, which, as noted earlier, can be delivered in institutions, in the home, or in such settings as supported housing. Some of these workers are paid while others are not. One category of paid workers, who have a variety of titles, such as personal support workers (PSWs) or health care aides, assist people with tasks that they would be able to do for themselves if they were not ill or disabled. These unregulated workers can work in a variety of settings (including LTC institutions, homes, and even hospitals), often under the supervision of registered nurses. In addition, a great deal of unpaid work is delivered by informal caregivers, often family members, who help people who have difficulty managing on their own. An ongoing policy debate concerns what sorts of supports these caregivers need and how best to provide these. The fiscal consequences can also be significant. Because difficulty in performing these ADL can be a major reason for people having to be admitted to nursing homes, even though remaining in their homes would be far less expensive, subsidizing the costs of home care can often save money.[8]

However, if they would otherwise have managed (alone or with unpaid helpers), then subsidizing their expenditures would represent an add-on. Accordingly, drawing the line about what should be publicly subsidized, and for whom, is usually far from simple; we will return to these issues in Chapters 7 and 8.

One consequence of professional regulation is that decisions about who will be registered to practise will depend on the jurisdiction. This gives rise to issues when people trained in one jurisdiction move into another and still want to practise their profession. This is a perennial problem for foreign-trained doctors and nurses. As will be noted in Chapter 4, health care in Canada is organized along provincial and territorial lines; that means these issues can arise even when health professionals move across provincial or territorial boundaries. However, the provincial and territorial colleges regulating each profession usually work together in national associations and have sought to standardize requirements and ease the ability of professionals registered in one province or territory to become registered should they move to another Canadian jurisdiction, although even this is not always smooth. One ongoing problem with telehealth programs, for example, is that the physician giving telehealth services needs to be registered in each province and territory where their patients are, which can make it very complex to deliver such services across jurisdictional boundaries.

Health Human Resources: How Many Do We Need?

Another ongoing issue is how many health care providers we need. Because it takes many years to train most health care providers, we cannot immediately create new supply. If you think of health human resources (HHR) as a stock of workers, then you can think of how we add to or subtract from this pool. New workers can be added in a number of ways, including new graduates from training programs, people immigrating to the jurisdiction, and existing workers deciding to work more hours or return to the labour force. They can be subtracted through death, retirement, emigration, or working fewer hours (including leaving to do other things). One key issue in HHR planning is sometimes called recruitment/retention – how do you convince people to work (and continue working) at a particular type of job (or, in a more fine-grained approach, in a particular subsector, geographical region, or organization). Clearly, workplaces vary in how successful they are at doing this. What has been called *stickiness* is the probability that someone working in a job (or, more broadly, in a sector or subsector of the workforce) will stay there the next year. In analysis of data about where Ontario nurses were working over time, we found considerable variation across nursing subsectors, with hospitals being highly sticky while home care was not.[9] Not surprisingly, recruitment and retention are affected by how well you treat (and pay) your workers. In the case of nursing, for example, job attractiveness is related to a host of factors, some financial (e.g., salary, benefits), some related to the ability to know when they would be working (working on a casual basis has been shown to be the least attractive to workers, who will often leave for jobs that offer them better benefits and more predictable working conditions), and many related to enjoying their work, having supportive colleagues, and feeling that they are helping patients.[10]

One policy question is who should be responsible for balancing supply and demand. If we attempt to plan ahead and project what the supply of workers and the demand or need for their services will be, we will have to successfully predict the future. This is notoriously difficult, and we rarely get it right. In market situations, this is irrelevant. If there are too many lawyers, some won't find work. This might be wasteful of their talent and energy, but it is not usually considered a public problem. If there are too few, then their earnings may go up – a delightful situation for those professionals, if not necessarily for those paying them or needing their services. However, health professionals are somewhat different, particularly since most people would agree that the consequences of not having them available when they are needed can be potentially serious. Issues related to how many we need and where they will practise are accordingly ongoing controversies, particularly given how long it takes to train new workers and the waste of their skills and training incurred if they are not employed. We could adopt a free rider model and not spend the money to train them; rather, we could hire them from other jurisdictions. This presents some serious ethical problems if the raided jurisdiction is then short of workers and also places residents of your own jurisdiction who want to enter those professions at a disadvantage. An additional complication arises when these workers are paid by taxpayers; they can be seen to represent both costs and benefits.

Another question is how much we should pay different workers. In turn, this question affects various approaches to cost constraint. One possibility is to use bargaining power (particularly if there is only one payer) to try to curb wages and benefits. However, this can lead to difficult labour relations, especially if the workers do not feel they are being fairly treated. For example, a number of provinces have been locked in disputes with their health care workers, particularly with physicians, about the fee schedules. Another possibility is labour substitution, where employers try to ensure that, where possible, work is done by lower paid workers (often under the supervision of other professionals). If physicians, who tend to be more highly paid, can work in a team with other professionals, the group may be able to see more patients for a lower cost. We may save money if midwives can handle uncomplicated childbirth instead of having to pay physicians to do this. Hospitals or LTC may replace some registered nurses (RNs) with lower paid licensed practical nurses (LPNs, sometimes called registered practical nurses or RPNs), or with non-registered PSWs. Self-care can move much of the burden of care to unpaid patients or their family members. This can be a win from a care point of view, although not for the professionals being displaced or paid less. Ironically, some of these efforts have evoked arguments about pay equity and the argument that if people are doing the same work, they should get the same pay. Ontario's midwives have made this argument and taken their case for being paid the same as GPs to the Human Rights Tribunal. Their argument is based on a 2013 report the midwives had commissioned from an independent pay equity expert, which concluded that midwives (the highest paid of whom were earning about

$100,000 annually to handle about 80 births per year) should be making 91% of what family physicians made (on average, $200,000). They are arguing that the reason for the difference is sex discrimination.[11] Others might argue that there are substantial differences in the training and activities of GPs and midwives, including in the number of patients they see. Certainly, accepting a pay equity argument would eliminate any cost-savings rationale for labour substitution.

As we will see, how health care services are paid for and delivered can vary considerably and will often depend on the type of service and on the characteristics of the person receiving them. Chapter 3 will examine the concept of insurance and markets, and clarify how different health systems reflect various combinations of public and private, and of financing and delivery. Chapter 4 will focus on how health care is financed and delivered in Canada. Chapter 5 will highlight several models that are used internationally and note how Canada compares. Together, these concepts will help our discussion of the second reform suggestion – improve care coordination and quality – in Chapter 8.

CHAPTER THREE

How Is Health Care Paid For and Delivered?

Economics studies how resources are distributed, with a focus on how markets work. (For those wanting greater detail, Hurley has written a well-regarded textbook on health economics.[1]) Since most people do not need health care most of the time, we will briefly describe the logic of insurance. We next examine health systems, focusing on two key concepts – the distinction between public and private, and the distinction between how care is paid for (financing) and how it is delivered. Note that precise details about how care is organized, delivered, and paid for may differ, not only across jurisdictions but also across the different types of services described in the previous chapter.

Insurance and How Health Care Differs From Other Goods and Services

Economics works on the assumption that markets attempt to balance supply and demand by using price signals. We can accordingly see how much I want something by how much I'm willing to pay for it. Prices should respond to demand to ensure that scarce goods go to those who value them the most. If supply is fixed, and demand is high, the price should go up until you are at the point where you balance supply and demand. For example, tickets for a playoff game or a concert by a popular band will become sufficiently expensive that those placing a lower value on seeing that event will drop out of the market, until all tickets are sold to those willing to pay the higher price. Conversely, if the price is free, demand should increase. If I am offered a free holiday trip for two, all expenses paid, at a time of my convenience, I and my chosen travel companion would probably go, even if I wouldn't have bought that ticket if I had to pay for it myself.

A related concept is that markets benefit from competition. These price signals assume not only that buyers will compete with other buyers but also that sellers will compete with one another for their business. Economic theory argues that perfect competition will thus ensure that resources move to where they are most needed and that prices will be lower, since those charging overly higher prices will find that others will be attracted into that market to compete with them by offering similar goods at lower prices.

Another widely used concept in economics is referred to as *moral hazard*. The idea originated from looking at the insurance industry; it argues that when people are protected from risks, they might behave in riskier ways because someone else will bear the costs. When applied to health care, these theorists argue that people would take advantage of free (or subsidized) goods, using them just because they are free. If true, it suggests that people should have to pay at least a token amount for items to ensure that resources are not being wasted.

Health care, however, doesn't always fit this economic model of supply and demand. The key distinction is the role of need. Economics deals with supply and demand; need does not play a role in markets except to the extent it influences demand. In contrast, for at least some health care goods and services, need replaces rather than influences demand. In a pure need-based model, if I need something, I should get it, and if I do not need it, I should not. For example, if I suddenly rupture my appendix and would have a high risk of dying unless I got treatment, most people would say that I should be treated, even if I don't have the money to pay for it. Conversely, if you offer me free open-heart surgery, I should not want it unless I need it. This contrasts to situations where supply and demand clearly do operate. For example, I may want a new pair of shoes, even if I have several good pairs already in my closet. If I can pay, most would agree that I should be able to buy them; if I can't, most would agree that I should not expect to receive them for free.

The distinction between health care and other services is not always black and white. One issue is knowledge; people may seek care because they are afraid they are ill, even if they are not. (They are sometimes called the *worried well*.) One obvious approach is better patient education, to help people know when they need care and when they do not. Unlike new shoes, there are few medical services that people want unless they believe they need them; even though I like my doctor, I can think of far more pleasant ways to spend time than waiting in her office for an unnecessary visit. However, moral hazard may be an issue for providers if they are in a payment model that gives them economic incentives to provide additional services. Fortunately, professionalism usually curbs these incentives; very few doctors would perform unnecessary surgery for the money, and those who do are usually caught by regulatory bodies and have their licence to practise removed.

An additional complication is that health care is often financed through insurance models. The logic of insurance is that people pool their costs to handle risks. With luck, lightning will not strike my house. However, if it does, and I have insurance, I will be able to cover the costs. Accordingly, those of us who avoid this catastrophe will be subsidizing the unlucky ones, in the knowledge that, should it have happened to us, we would have been subsidized by the other members of that insurance pool. For insurance models to be stable, it is critical that the total revenues available (which would usually result from the premiums charged to plan members, plus the return on investment of that money) be set high enough to cover the expected costs to be paid out (which include the costs of running the insurance plan).

If we use an insurance model, there are a number of ways to set the premiums that people must pay into the pool. One possibility is to set flat rates, with everyone paying the same. Another is to base the premiums on ability to pay, which means the wealthier are subsidizing those with less money. The most common approach is to base the premiums on the costs the person is expected to generate, sometimes called *actuarial fairness*. These may be risk rated (based on the expected costs of services required) or be based on various other factors, including age-sex group, income, or employment status. We may also decide that certain people are so high risk that we don't want them in our risk pool. If you have built your house on a flood plain, we may not want to sell you flood insurance. If you have a terrible driving record, we will almost certainly charge you higher rates, and at some point, we may say that you can no longer drive (and certainly that we won't sell you automobile insurance). And you emphatically cannot insure against a certainty; in that case, it is no longer insurance. I cannot buy insurance for my house after it has burned down. In a pure insurance model, some would therefore argue that you should not have complete coverage, or moral hazard may set in. You don't want to give me an incentive to total my car so that I can get a nice new one or to burn down my business if it is no longer profitable so that I can collect the insurance.

Clearly, health care doesn't really fit this logic very well. Should a pregnant woman be able to purchase insurance to cover birth and delivery? The logic of insurance would say no, even though most of us would agree that it is preferable to ensure that people do not have to give birth without proper assistance. Similarly, if I have a history of cancer, should I be ousted from the insurance pool? Private insurance often works that way – if I have a pre-existing condition, I may not be able to get coverage for it. Most people would agree, however, that it would be both foolish and inhumane to deny people already dealing with a serious illness insurance coverage for the costs arising from treating it.

Some health insurance models do try to follow these insurance principles. In an effort to reduce moral hazard and discourage people from unnecessary visits, for example, many insurance plans in many countries make those who receive services pay some of the cost. These user fees can take several forms, which are not mutually exclusive. A *co-payment* means that the person receiving care must pay a fixed amount of each bill. For example, if you see your doctor, you might be required to pay $20 per visit, with your insurance paying the rest. Co-insurance computes the user fee as a percentage of the bill; for example, 20% co-insurance means that your insurance will pay 80% of the bill, and you will pay the remaining 20%. Another approach is for the insurance not to begin until the recipient has paid a certain sum, often called a deductible. Depending on the plan, full coverage may begin once the person's payments have exceeded that amount, or the person may still be responsible for co-pays or co-insurance. There may also be a limit on how much a plan will cover (particularly for private insurance), with the patient responsible for all costs that exceed that cap. Conversely, plans may set an out-of-pocket maximum, after which the insurer will pick up 100% of the eligible costs. There can be considerable variation across systems, insurance plans, and even types of care. As we will see in Chapter 4, Canada employs *first dollar coverage* without any co-pays or deductibles for all medically necessary physician and hospital services, but not necessarily for other services. In Ontario, for example, the Ontario Drug Benefit covers some of the drug costs for those over age 65, but at the time of writing it charged a deductible of $100, plus a per-prescription co-payment of "up to $6.11" for each approved prescription drug; these fees could be reduced, or waived, for qualifying low-income seniors.[2] (Some pharmacies are known to reduce these fees in order to attract more customers.) Co-payments for dental or vision care, which are almost entirely privately funded in Canada, can be even higher.

To better analyse how different health care systems can operate, it is helpful to clarify the difference between public and private, the difference between financing and delivery, and how these come together into health care systems.

Public versus Private, and Financing versus Delivery

It is important to distinguish between how services are paid for (financing) and how they are delivered. In that connection, the terms *public* and *private* can apply to both how care is financed and how it is delivered. A further complication is that both public and private can be subdivided into several categories.[3] Public refers to government, which in turn can have various levels, such as national; provincial, territorial, or state; regional; and local. Private can include corporate for-profit business (which has a responsibility to maximize return to its shareholders); for-profit small business (which may include health care professional practices, such as physician or physiotherapist offices, a category Canadian health economist Robert Evans calls "not only for profit"); not-for-profit (NFP) organizations (which can be large, such as many hospitals, or small, such as some community agencies); and individuals and their families (who may pay for or provide many services). To this can be added quasi-public organizations, which are legally private but heavily regulated and thus span the boundary between public and private. Examples of the quasi-public category include many of the Canadian regional health authorities described in Chapter 4 and many of the European sickness funds that provide health care insurance. How close these various bodies are to being public clearly varies, depending on how they have been set up. For example, depending on the province, the regional health authorities may be incorporated as private non-profit bodies (which would put them officially in the private category), but may have boards who are appointed by government (which would make them closer to being public); some people prefer to use the term *public arm's-length organizations*.

If we look at how health care services are delivered, we can classify providers into various categories along the public-private continuum. A government-owned hospital would be classified as public delivery; this has been a common model in such countries as England, Australia, and Sweden, as well as for military hospitals in the United States and other countries. Hospitals in Canada largely fall into the private NFP category, although in many provinces (but not in Ontario), they have been subsumed into regional health authorities, which usually fall into the quasi-public category. Physician offices in many jurisdictions are classified private for-profit small businesses (although, since these usually fall into the "not only for profit" category, they are expected to also look out for the best interests of their patients rather than only trying to maximize their incomes). Pharmaceutical companies are usually private for-profit investor-owned corporations. Note that many combinations are possible, particularly as countries experiment with alternative ways of delivering care.

Policy analysts use the term *privatization* to refer to the movement from public to private. This can include changes both in how things are financed and in how they are delivered. For example, some jurisdictions have been transferring formerly government-owned enterprises to the private sector; examples include transportation (e.g., selling off formerly government-owned railroads) and even prisons, which are privately run in some jurisdictions outside Canada. A major trend towards privatization, or partial privatization, of some activities has developed over the last decade in a wide range of countries, including the United Kingdom, France, Canada, and New Zealand. A related example is the use of public-private partnerships (sometimes called P3s) where private sector businesses participate with government in the delivery of infrastructure or services that had traditionally been provided by governments alone, usually with a guarantee of public financing.

The Organisation for Economic Co-operation and Development (OECD) is an international organization with 34 member countries, whose mandate is to compare and coordinate policy proposals and use "its wealth of information on a broad range of topics to help governments foster prosperity and fight poverty through economic growth and financial stability. We help ensure the environmental implications of economic and social development are taken into account."[4] (We will examine its rankings of different health systems, and where Canada is placed, in Chapter 5.)

To make it simpler to compare systems, the OECD has classified the many ways to finance health and social services into four main categories. All these categories are being used in Canada, albeit for different categories of people and services. The first category is entirely public; the money may come from general revenues or from special taxes or premiums that are officially designated as being for health care. That is how Canada finances physician and hospital services. The second category, which falls into the public or quasi-public category, uses a social insurance model (usually with compulsory membership) whereby government and/or some heavily regulated quasi-public organizations run an insurance system. In Canada and the United States, publicly financed old-age pensions often use this model, whereby all working people and their employers must contribute to

the pool and then can draw on it to collect pensions once they retire. The third funding model relies on private third-party insurance,
which is a major source of funding for such services as pharmaceuticals, vision care, and dental care for those Canadians with private
coverage. The fourth funding model is also private but uses direct
out-of-pocket payments from the person receiving the services; this
is used by those Canadians without private insurance to pay for those
services not covered by public insurance.

As one example, Owen Adams and Sharon Vanin analysed options
for paying for LTC in Canada. Their suggestions for ways to do this
came from all of these four categories: it could be financed through
general tax revenues, social insurance (with contributions from employers and employees), privately purchased LTC insurance, and private savings.[5]

Putting the dimensions of financing and delivery and public and
private together makes it clear that health care systems (or components of them) can represent various combinations of public and private and financing and delivery. Different models can be used not
only in different jurisdictions but also for different categories of services and clients, which extend beyond health care.[6] The OECD's terminology is shown in the two-by-two classification in Table 3.1.

The public financing-public delivery cell, which the OECD calls a
"public-integrated model," includes services that are paid for publicly
and where the people who work in them are deemed to be public servants or employees. As we will see in Chapter 5, the UK National
Health Service (NHS) largely falls into this cell. In Canada few health
care services fall into this category, with the exception of public
health and, in some provinces, government-run provincial psychiatric
hospitals (although almost all of them have been shifted to private
NFP status). A common non-health example that falls into this cell is
public schools, where the teachers are paid by, and work for, public
school boards.

The private financing-public delivery cell (which the OECD does
not even bother to label) is widely believed to be suboptimal for health
care and plays a minimal part in most developed countries, although
it is still used in many developing countries that do not have the resources to publicly cover even medically necessary services. However,

3.1 Classification of health care systems

	Public financing	Private financing
Public delivery	public-integrated model	(user fees for public services)
Private delivery	public contract model	private insurance/provider model

this category is used for other types of services. For example, in most countries, including Canada, much public transit would fall into that classification, since it is delivered by people working for government (usually at the local level) but is largely funded privately (in the case of transit, through the fare box).

In Canada the hospital and physician services falling under the *Canada Health Act* (discussed in Chapter 4) largely fall into the public financing-private delivery cell that the OECD calls "public contracting"; the providers are private, but the money comes largely from public sources. If we consider social insurance as being public financing (or at least quasi-public financing), then, as noted in Chapter 5, Germany would also be an example of this cell.

Finally, services in the private financing-private delivery cell are delivered by private providers and paid for privately (either by the user of that service or by private insurance). In Canada a number of services, including dental care, vision care, much rehabilitation, and some outpatient pharmaceuticals, as well as those physician services which are not deemed medically necessary (e.g., cosmetic surgery) fall into this cell.

Note that the United States has multiple models, which fall into most of the cells of Table 3.1. For example, the Veteran's Administration would be classified as public financing-public delivery, while the US Medicare/Medicaid programs would be classified as public financing-private delivery, and most of the care received by those with private insurance (as well as those with no insurance at all) would fall into the private financing-private delivery category. In Chapter 5 we will consider the United States to be an example of the private financing-private delivery category.

Which model is best? Internationally, there is considerable variation in the mix of funding approaches that are used; these may also vary across type of service and category of client.[7] Considerable research has been conducted on the relative efficiency and effectiveness of the private and public sectors in meeting health and social objectives.[8] One thing that was clear is that the devil is in the details. Different funding models also reflect different views about which costs should be born collectively and which should be the responsibility of individuals and their families. All services are not the same. One useful way to distinguish between different kinds of services, and hence the extent to which competition is likely to be helpful, is by looking at what analysts refer to as their *production characteristics*.[9]

One of these production characteristics, sometimes called *contestability*, refers to the barriers to entering and exiting a market. These might include high sunk costs associated with such activities as building and maintaining the necessary facilities and acquiring highly specialized expertise. Contestability is low when these barriers to entry and exit are high. Thus, Walmart may decide to compete with local pharmacies by selling over-the-counter drugs, since anyone already working for their stores would be able to ring up the purchases. It is much less likely to decide it wants to open a pediatric heart surgery unit to compete with the local children's hospital. Clearly, it is easier to have a competitive market when contestability is high.

Another production characteristic is *measurability*, which deals with how easy it is to measure what is being done. Again, different goods and services vary in their measurability. It is relatively simple to judge whether a laboratory test has been done correctly; we can just send a sample and see whether the lab gets the right results. It is much harder to measure whether a family practitioner listens to her patients (or indeed, whether a childcare worker truly loves the children she is caring for). Simple metrics, such as the number of hugs per hour, recorded on a wall chart, are unlikely to capture these important but difficult-to-measure elements. Again, competition is easier when measurability is high; otherwise we don't know whether important corners are being cut.

Another production characteristic is (somewhat misleadingly) called *complexity*. It does not refer to how complex the activity is but to whether the activity stands on its own or needs to be integrated with other activities. As an example, if a hospital needs a laboratory test in the middle of the night, it is not helpful to have contracted out all their tests to an off-site facility that is only open from 9 to 5 on Monday through Friday.

When performance standards and goals are easily specified and where programs are amenable to explicit arm's-length monitoring and control (i.e., when measurability is high), private for-profit delivery can be efficient, although other forms of delivery may also perform well. However, when there are multiple goals, the benefits of encouraging provision by the for-profit private sector are less clear, particularly when there is a risk that other desired outcomes could be sacrificed to improve profitability. One obvious example is when certain populations are more, or less, profitable to serve. International evidence clearly demonstrates that for-profit hospitals are less willing to serve people without good health insurance, regardless of those people's clinical needs. Such people are then either served by other organizations (which could be public or NFP hospitals), or are not served at all (with the possible exception of emergency cases that need immediate management or stabilization).

Another important nuance is the balance between competition and cooperation. This becomes particularly important when we seek to integrate services, since it is unlikely that an organization will want to cooperate with one of its rivals. This has been an ongoing issue in the United States, where competing health insurance plans often place limits on the ability of their clients to receive insured health care services from providers who are not part of their network. Cooperation tends to be easier when the organizations don't have a responsibility to maximize the return to their shareholders.

To make things even more complex, regardless of who is paying, providers can be paid in a number of ways. This concept is sometimes termed *allocation*; it deals with how resources flow from payers to providers and the different incentives that go with different payment models. In turn, as noted below, payment models influence what providers have incentive to do (or not do). One categorization of approaches to paying providers uses two dimensions.[10] The first dimension is whether payment goes directly from the payers to the individual providers or whether payment goes to provider organizations (e.g., hospitals, primary care organizations), who then pay the providers. One aspect of recent efforts to reform primary care has been the movement of physicians from solo-practice models into these kinds of provider organizations, which may then have more flexibility as to which providers they employ and how they pay them. It is accordingly important to recognize that the money that providers receive from a payer (including government-run health insurance plans) is usually not the same as a salary. Depending on the model, these payments are expected to cover the overhead costs (including the costs of renting, heating, and maintaining the space, buying equipment, and paying staff). This can become particularly misleading when government payers are battling physicians about fee schedules and implying that their billings equate to their take-home pay.

The second dimension of payment models is the basis of payment. A number of approaches can be used, alone or in combination (sometimes called *blended models*). Providers can be paid for actual costs (e.g., drug plans could reimburse for the actual costs of pharmaceuticals plus a mark-up). They can be paid for time spent (e.g., wages, fixed payments for someone to work a particular shift). They can be reimbursed for each service they provide, using such methods as fee-for-service (FFS) or activity-based funding. They can be paid based on the population they serve, often on the basis of capitation, which gives a fixed payment, potentially adjusted for such characteristics as age, sex, and how ill a person is, for each person on their roster. They can get bonus payments for achieving particular goals (e.g., pay for performance). They could also receive a fixed or global budget (which is often based on historical spending levels); this is how hospitals have traditionally been paid in Canada.

Economists often decompose total costs into *fixed costs*, which are required to run a service and tend to remain the same regardless of how many services are being produced (the output), and *variable costs*, which change as the number of units being produced changes. These fixed costs may also include quasi-fixed costs, which are essentially fixed up to a certain volume of production but require additional resources if the volume increases beyond that level. (Accountants make a similar but not identical distinction between capital costs and operating costs, which is less useful for this purpose, since it does not really pick up the difference between operating costs that are fixed and those that vary with the number of services provided.) For many services, there are also *economies of scale*, where the average cost of providing a service decreases with service volume. One example is the costs to run a public school. There are fixed costs to build, heat, and maintain the building, regardless of how many students attend. There are also quasi-fixed costs for each classroom (including the costs of paying a teacher), which will jump if enrolment becomes large enough that another classroom needs to be staffed. There are small variable costs that will increase with enrolment, such as purchasing textbooks. If reimbursement is based only on average costs, some obvious problems can arise. For example, when fixed costs and quasi-fixed costs (e.g., rent, salaries) are a relatively high proportion of the total costs, then service-based funding models have the potential for perverse incentives because the variable costs of having more, or fewer, students are smaller than the average costs incorporated into the funding formula. These perverse incentives can take multiple forms. For example, a service-based funding model will underpay in most rural or remote areas, where a school must be staffed even if relatively few students are available to use it. Conversely, service-based models may overpay facilities that can attract additional students as long as they can be handled by the existing infrastructure. Similar problems may arise in trying to fund hospitals, physicians, and other health care services on an average-cost basis.

One reason that the basis for payment makes a difference is that different payment models have different incentive structures.[11] For example, from a purely economic viewpoint, and recognizing that providers also seek to meet the needs of their patients, global budgets give an incentive to do as little as possible to ensure that the budget is not exceeded; FFS gives an incentive to deliver more services to increase revenues; and capitation gives an incentive to select the lowest cost clients (and then to do as little for them as possible, only keeping them happy enough to retain them as clients). The appropriate model thus depends both on the cost structures involved and on the desired patterns of servicing.

Funding models are hence a perennial target for change, and history has shown that there is rarely a right answer. Historically, Canada tended to pay its hospitals based on global budgets, and pay its doctors FFS, although these models are both changing as payers seek to react to the weaknesses of each payment method. Many provinces are thus trying to move their hospitals to activity-based funding, which pays on the basis of what services are being done (much like FFS), and at the same time trying to move their physicians away from FFS to capitated-funding models. Not surprisingly, they are finding that they then move from having to deal with the weaknesses of the older funding model to having to deal with the weaknesses of the method they have chosen to replace it. The current trend is for blended models in the hope that a good compromise can be reached.

One approach is to tie payment models to the characteristics needed to ensure a high-quality, high-performing health system, with particular attention to whether there is overuse, underuse, or misuse of the particular services.[12] For example, if there was underuse of some important services, FFS would provide incentives to ensure that more would be provided. However, if there was already overuse, the incentives might make things worse; in that case, a model such as global funding might provide incentives to do less.

Fortunately, these fiscal incentives to over- or under-provide services are often balanced by professionalism. As professionals, health care providers are expected to ensure that appropriate care is given, even if this would not maximize their profits. They are not expected to withhold care even if global budgeting would encourage underservice; neither are they expected to recommend unnecessary care to collect additional fees. However, most agree that it seems unwise to design incentives so that the best providers are punished financially for behaving professionally.

The choice of payment mechanisms is also related to views about government roles versus the role of the market, which in turn is related to views about what type of good health care is seen to be. For example, even if I do not use a hospital emergency room, I still benefit from what economists call the *option value* of having it available should I need it, but if care is paid for only by those actually receiving services (as opposed to being at least partially financed through tax revenues), there is no obvious way to make me pay for that option value, since I would not be using that service as long as I stay healthy.

One way to look at how we might want to pay for health care services is to sort these services into four categories (which we called "flavours" in a paper), each of which presents somewhat different policy issues.[13]

The first flavour refers to public health services for the entire population, including ensuring clean air and clean water, and protection against infectious diseases. For the most part, these services are likely to meet the definition of public goods described in Chapter 1 and hence probably should be paid for by government.

The second flavour covers basic health care to individuals, where anticipated costs are small and relatively homogeneous. This may include basic visits to family doctors or certain types of common and relatively inexpensive medications (e.g., pills to lower blood pressure). In theory, this category of care could be seen as similar to housing and food; like them, it could be paid for by the individuals receiving these services, with some public subsidy to help people who might have trouble covering the costs. Sometimes leaving these costs to be covered by individuals, risking that people will not use those services if they are short of money, might save some money in the short term but cost far more in the long run. As an example, suppose people have debilitating and expensive strokes because they could not afford the relatively inexpensive medications needed to control their blood pressure. However, similar arguments could be made about people who become ill because they cannot afford food or shelter. We could accordingly justify treating these costs in much the same way as other social welfare programs; we could also – and most countries do – justify including them within a universal health insurance model.

The third flavour includes potentially catastrophically expensive services to individuals, where costs are skewed but not predictable; this is precisely what insurance is designed to cover. An example might be a person badly injured in an automobile accident or people who get a serious disease even though they were not known to be at high risk for it.

The fourth flavour includes potentially catastrophically expensive services to high-risk individuals, where we know that these costs are both high and very likely to occur. One example is someone who already has a disease and knows they will need to continue to take expensive medications. Those people are not attractive candidates for voluntary risk pools, particularly in competitive markets, and hence may find themselves unable to purchase insurance for the care they need.

This analysis suggests that the policies about how to finance and deliver one category of services to one segment of the population may not necessarily work well for others.

The next chapter will take a closer look at how Canada has organized and financed health care.

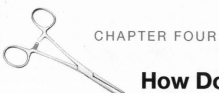

CHAPTER FOUR

How Does Canada Do It?

How Our System of Government Affects Health Care (Federal, Provincial, Territorial)

There is an old joke about an international competition to write a book about elephants. The submissions play on various national stereotypes. For example, the French are said to have written about the love life of the elephant and the Germans to have prepared a comprehensive 12-volume encyclopedia about elephants. The Canadian entry was *The Elephant: A Federal or Provincial Responsibility?* Certainly, far too often, discussions about how to achieve particular goals end up in a discussion of whose responsibility it is.

Canada, like many other countries, is a federation, with a national government (the federal government) and a series of sub-national jurisdictions (provinces and territories). Such federations are always a balancing act. Which things should be standardized across the country, and which should be left to sub-national jurisdictions? How much local variation is acceptable? When Canada was formed in 1867, its neighbour to the south had just emerged from a civil war. One of the many ways of interpreting this war was as a battle about the relationships between the national government and its sub-national units (which the United States called states), and the extent to which national goals can (and should) prevail over local views. Accordingly, Canada's Fathers of Confederation thought it critically important to clarify what the powers of these two levels of government would be.

Amending Canada's Constitution has proven very difficult. Accordingly, what was then called the *British North America Act*, and subsequently renamed the *Constitution Act*,[1] set the rules that still guide the division of powers in Canada. This legislation, first enacted in 1867, gave the national government power over everything the Fathers of Confederation thought would be expensive or of national interest, and left the things deemed less expensive or for which variation across jurisdictions would seem appropriate to the provinces. To further complicate matters, Canada also has three large but sparsely populated northern territories, whose roles and powers officially fall under federal jurisdiction, albeit with much of this delegated to their own territorial governments. Accordingly, the distribution of powers between the federal and provincial governments described in this chapter do not formally apply to the territories, although in practice the federal government may (or may not) chose to apply similar policies. Certain populations also have separate arrangements. For example, First Nations living on reserves were designated as a federal rather than provincial responsibility (with provisions for self-government). Members of the armed services, who could be killed or injured in service to their country, were recognized as being entitled to some services to be paid for by the federal government. (One consequence is that people can fall through the cracks as the different payers argue about whose responsibility that person is; this has been a particular problem for First Nations.) This volume will focus primarily on the federal and provincial or territorial levels, with little emphasis on the special provisions for such groups as First Nations, which could be the subject of another book.

Section 91 of the Constitution listed the responsibilities given to the federal government. One of these was "Quarantine and the Establishment and Maintenance of Marine Hospitals"; another was the ability to raise money "by any Mode or System of Taxation" which gave it considerable "spending power." The national government was also given the residual power to legislate for the "peace, order, and good government of Canada" on any matters not assigned to the provinces.

. The provisions in the Constitution were based on the realities of life in 1867. Determining what currency Canada would use, or what systems of weights and measures, was made a federal responsibility so that the individual provinces/territories could not decide to set up their own currencies. As noted above, other things were designated as national responsibilities because they were expensive or because they were important to nation building; at the time, this was defined as items such as canals and railroads. What was inexpensive at the time, and hence left as a provincial responsibility, included local governments, which were given no official role in Canada's Constitution. Cities and regions within a province are thus creatures of their province, and their powers (and boundaries) can be changed by their provincial governments should those governments be willing to pay the electoral consequences. Among the provincial responsibilities listed in section 92 of the Constitution were "The Establishment, Maintenance, and Management of Hospitals, Asylums, Charities, and Eleemosynary Institutions in and for the Province, other than Marine Hospitals" and "Generally all Matters of a merely local or private Nature in the Province." Although few realized it at the time, these provisions have proven critical in determining who would have responsibility for health care in Canada.

In 1867 the great advances of medicine were in the future. Many hospitals were still charitable institutions where sick people went when their home was not nice enough, rather than places that might cure you, although Florence Nightingale was beginning to change this in England and eventually internationally. But from that brief mention of hospitals in section 92, subsequent court decisions interpreted those clauses as placing most of health care under provincial jurisdiction. The provinces also had control over education and professional licensure; that means that health professionals must be registered within a province or territory rather than at the national level. As noted in Chapter 2, one modern implication of these provisions from 1867 is that telehealth cannot provide professional services across provincial or territorial boundaries unless those providing them are licensed in every province and territory they are serving.

Constitutional responsibility for other parts of health care, particularly health protection and public health, is more ambiguous. The federal government was given responsibility for "quarantine," but once people had disembarked from their boats, they (and their health care) were deemed to be a provincial responsibility. The Canadian compromise has been to give provincial governments jurisdiction over most public health activities; this usually includes such things as sanitation, public health, and the prevention of communicable diseases. In turn, they can (and often do) devolve this to local governments. This distribution of powers perhaps made some sense when "around the world in 80 days" was a major accomplishment but can be problematic when epidemic diseases can quickly leap across boundaries. Whereas in the past those already infected with a disease would usually become ill on the voyage, they may now arrive while they still seem healthy and unwittingly spread the infection after their arrival. (SARS was one example, where the person who spread it in Ontario had not travelled abroad; he was the son of a woman who contracted it in China in 2003, become ill two days after returning home to Toronto, and infected her son before she died at home of what was then thought to be cardiac failure.[2]) One possible way of giving authority to the federal government is to rely on the federal power over criminal law and international trade; this has been used to give the federal government some authority to pass legislation to prevent the transmission of a "public evil" that is determined to be a danger to public health (examples of legislation include the *Food and Drugs Act* and the *Hazardous Products Act*). However, the scope of this power is limited.

Another way in which the federal government may be granted jurisdiction over health-related matters is if these are deemed to fall under the auspices of the justice system. For example, when the Supreme Court of Canada ruled that prohibiting medically assisted deaths was a violation of Canada's *Charter of Rights and Freedoms*, their decision moved this from being a matter for health care providers only (and hence falling under provincial jurisdiction) to falling at least partially under federal jurisdiction. This has forced the federal government to pass new legislation about when and under what conditions such assisted deaths should be permitted, which is still being heatedly debated at the time of writing. Related disputes have concerned whether policies about substance abuse (e.g., needle exchange programs, safe injection sites) fell under the criminal justice system (which would make them a federal responsibility) or were counted as health care (which would make them a provincial responsibility). The courts ruled that it was an example of health, which made it a provincial matter and meant that the federal government of the day could not close down the BC needle exchange program for drug users.

Views about the appropriate role for government have also changed over time. In 1867 neither education nor health care were generally seen as public responsibilities. However, as noted in Chapter 5, in the twentieth century, many countries (including Germany and England) came under pressure to take on a greater government role in such social services as health care and pensions. This pressure was accentuated by the need for support for veterans of World War I and their families, and a belief that the government had some responsibility to those who had been hurt in service to their country. The same pressures affected Canada. Another rationale in Canada was the expansion of settlement by European immigrants, particularly into the Prairie provinces. The federal government had used its powers to encourage this expansion through building railroads. However, as Canada welcomed these new immigrants, it also recognized the difficulties in providing medical care to those leaving the cities to settle other parts of the country and that successful settlement of these areas would be aided by ensuring that medical care would still be available to those moving there. Since health care was deemed a provincial responsibility, some provinces did move to fill this gap. Saskatchewan allowed local communities to hire municipal doctors on contract. Saskatchewan and Alberta established "union hospital districts" in some rural communities, whereby the local municipalities and towns worked together to provide (and pay for) running local hospitals. Similarly, Newfoundland set up publicly run cottage hospitals. Other charitable organizations, including the Red Cross, were also active in helping ensure health care services would be available in certain communities.

One problem soon became evident; there was considerable difference in how wealthy the different provinces were and hence in how much each could afford to do. This problem is not unique to Canada. Most federal systems must decide how to deal with differences in the economic capacity of their component parts. One key question that arises is what it means to be a citizen (or resident) of a country, as opposed to being a resident of a particular sub-national (or local) jurisdiction, in terms of the sorts of services people are entitled to. When is it important to ensure that everyone living in that nation has access to roughly equal levels of certain services, regardless of where they happen to be living and the ability of that region to pay for these services? Conversely, when can service levels be allowed to vary to match local needs and priorities? Jurisdictions vary in which services are seen as requiring national standards. In general, in most countries, health care and education are usually seen as requiring minimum national standards, although richer jurisdictions can exceed these should they (and their voters) choose. However, in Canada, both health and education fall under provincial and territorial jurisdiction, which presented problems for the less wealthy provinces and territories. Another issue, which arose periodically, was the incentive for one jurisdiction to deal with people needing care by encouraging them to move to a more generous jurisdiction. (On occasion, this involved buying them one-way bus or train tickets.) This was not well received by the receiving communities and came with the risk of leading to a race to the bottom. Setting national standards for what was deemed an appropriate minimum level of service seemed to be one way of dealing with such potential problems. In turn, this meant that mechanisms would have to be developed to ensure that all jurisdictions were able to pay for these agreed-on service levels.

One response used by many countries, including Canada, has been what is often called *fiscal federalism*; this approach uses a variety of mechanisms for transferring resources from the national government to its sub-national jurisdictions to help equalize their fiscal capacity and thereby allow (at least in theory) all communities to have sufficient resources to allow them to provide roughly comparable levels of services. (Provinces and territories may also use similar approaches to try to equalize the fiscal capacity of local communities within their jurisdiction.)

The formulas that are used vary. Two main approaches that Canada has used are cash grants and tax room (also called tax points). *Cash grants* are direct transfers from one level of government to another. *Tax room* refers to an agreement whereby the senior level of government decreases its tax rate, leaving room for the sub-national units to increase their tax rates (should they choose to do so) without increasing the total tax burden on the individual taxpayer. Note that tax points cannot be taken back; if the federal government decides to increase its tax rate, it has no mechanism to compel provincial or territorial governments to lower theirs. Unlike cash payments, tax points also do not give the senior level of government any power to enforce how the resulting resources are used. How much revenue tax points can yield is also related to the economic health of a particular jurisdiction; if residents do not have much taxable income, then tax points cannot yield much revenue. In contrast, cash grants can be tied to terms and conditions, and withheld should those conditions be violated.

The total amount of funds that will be transferred through these formulas can also vary. In Canada the formula is often based on combinations of how much is being spent on programs, the population of each jurisdiction (which may or may not be adjusted to weight the amount payable to take into account such factors as age distribution, perceived needs of different groups, etc.), and differences in fiscal capacity across jurisdictions. In Canada as in many federal states, these arrangements have long been contentious, since different models give rise to different winners and losers.

When Canada revised its Constitution in 1982, it included a provision under subsection 36(2) that "Parliament and the government of Canada are committed to the principle of making equalization payments to ensure that provincial governments have sufficient revenues to provide reasonably comparable levels of public services at reasonably comparable levels of taxation." This provision was implemented through a number of federal programs for transferring revenue to the provinces and territories. At the time of writing, Canada had four main transfer programs: the Canada Health Transfer (CHT), the Canada Social Transfer (CST), Equalization, and Territorial Formula Financing (which applies only to the three northern territories).[3] Although the precise formulas and conditions have varied over time, as will be noted below, at present these transfers are largely unconditional and simply go into provincial or territorial government general revenues.

Financing Health Care in Canada

Approaches to financing health care in Canada have evolved over time, and, as noted above, have used a variety of mechanisms.[4] Plans for government-funded health insurance were galvanized by the depression and World War II. In general, Saskatchewan led the way. The emphasis on settling the west had caused the population to grow rapidly; the census estimated it had grown from 91,279 people in 1901 to 895,992 by 1941, most of whom lived in the southern half of the province. In 1944 they had elected a social democratic government – the first democratic socialist government in North America. Its leader, Tommy Douglas (whom a Canada-wide survey designated as "The Greatest Canadian" in 2004), was committed to ensuring that all residents of the province would have access to hospital care. His government started in 1944 by providing funds to assist with the capital construction of hospitals.

In 1945, the federal government suggested, in what was called the Green Book Proposals, that there should be federal-provincial cooperation to develop a national program for social security, which would include health insurance. Not surprisingly, this cooperation was difficult to achieve, and the Green Book Proposals were never implemented. However, in 1948, the federal government (under Prime Minister Mackenzie King) did adopt a similar program to Saskatchewan's, providing cash payments to provincial and territorial governments for selected programs (e.g., hospital construction), using a program called the National Health Grants program. (To Saskatchewan's dismay, since the program was intended to build new hospitals, the province did not qualify for federal support for most of the hospitals it had already built.[5])

Meanwhile, Saskatchewan took the next step to help ensure that its population would have access to health services. In 1947 the provincial government introduced the single-payer Saskatchewan Hospital Services Plan, the first universal hospital insurance program in North America. Two other western provinces, British Columbia and Alberta, soon followed Saskatchewan's initiative. This put increasing pressure on the federal government to help with the costs.

In 1957 the federal government of Prime Minister Louis St-Laurent acted, passing the *Hospital Insurance and Diagnostic Services Act* (HIDS) with all-party approval. HIDS provided federal funds to the provinces and territories to cover about half the costs of their publicly funded hospital insurance programs (should they choose to have one) as long as they complied with national conditions. (The formula was more complex than a simple cost-shared model, since the amount the federal government contributed was based on a combination of the amount spent by that province and the average amount spent across the country.) The HIDS model did not provide federal funds for those activities that were seen as clearly provincial responsibilities (and were already being done by at least some provincial governments); accordingly, mental hospitals and tuberculosis sanatoria were not eligible for cost sharing under HIDS. Provinces did not have to set up a qualifying publicly funded hospital insurance plan, but the political pressure from their voters to do so became intense, particularly since they would only have to pay about half the costs and because it was hard to justify why their residents were paying (through their federal taxes) for similar programs in other provinces without receiving any benefits themselves. When HIDS began on July 1, 1958, only five provinces (Newfoundland, Manitoba, Saskatchewan, Alberta, and British Columbia) had set up hospital insurance programs, but all provinces were participating by January 1961.

In 1962 Saskatchewan promptly took the money it was saving because of the federal contributions and set up a single-payer universal insurance program to cover physician services. Douglas was no longer premier (he had become leader of the federal New Democratic Party), but the province continued his policy legacy. Saskatchewan's doctors were not impressed; they promptly went on strike to block socialized medicine. The strike lasted about 23 days. Its consequences, although serious, were less severe than they might have been, both because the province brought in some replacement doctors (from the United Kingdom) and, according to some sources, because some of the striking doctors, as ethical professionals, undermined their protest by continuing to see their sick patients who needed their care. Following mediation by Lord Stephen Taylor of the United Kingdom, a compromise was reached; there would indeed be a universal single-payer government-run insurance plan in Saskatchewan, but the physicians would not be salaried employees of government. Instead, they would continue to be independent professionals and would be paid largely on a FFS basis. This model of physicians as private providers who received their funding from a government-run single payer (the public funding-private delivery model described in Chapter 3) has remained a cornerstone of health care in Canada.

At the same time, a national examination of health care was underway. Again, Saskatchewan's influence was profound. In June 1961 Canada's Conservative Prime Minister John Diefenbaker, who was born in Ontario but grew up in and was elected from Saskatchewan asked Justice Emmett Hall to chair a Royal Commission on Health Services that would look closely at health care in Canada and make recommendations on how to ensure "that the best possible health care is available to all Canadians." The Hall Commission's final report was published in 1964. Hall, a member of the Conservative Party, had also lived in Saskatchewan and had served as chief justice of Saskatchewan before being appointed to the Supreme Court of Canada. The commission did a thorough job, hearing from hundreds of witnesses. When the report was released, Liberal Lester Pearson (from Ontario, without the Saskatchewan connection) had replaced Diefenbaker as prime minister. To the surprise of many, the Hall Report recommended that Saskatchewan's model should be adopted nationally, arguing that providing health care was cheaper than allowing people to have unnecessary illnesses.

In 1966 the federal government took the next step to implement the Hall Report's recommendations, passing the *Medical Care Act*; this legislation provided new federal cost sharing to any provinces that wanted to set up universal single-payer provincial insurance plans for medically necessary physician services. Again, this law galvanized provincial action; by 1971 all provinces had set up complying plans. Unlike with the NHS model in England, Canada retained its private-provider model. Government insurance plans paid many of the costs for private (albeit often NFP) delivery by the existing providers, using the public contracting model described in Chapter 3.

The way in which Canada's Constitution divided power, and the way it introduced its methods for cost sharing health care financing with the provinces, has had an enormous impact on how health care in Canada is financed and delivered. Since these models cost-shared only for hospital and physician services, any community-based care provided by non-physicians was not eligible for federal matching funds. The provinces thus had strong incentives to focus their models of health care delivery on hospitals and doctors, even if other approaches might have been more cost-efficient. That was one reason that the nurse practitioner program in Burlington, Ontario, although very successful clinically,[6] did not succeed at that time; for the program to get federal money, the patients in those clinics would also have to be seen by a physician, even if the nurse practitioner had already treated them. Similarly, there was no incentive for provincial health plans to move care out of hospitals unless the savings would be large enough to compensate for their loss of federal funds. As a result, Canadian health care had little incentive to shift to more cost-effective ways of delivering services.

Recognizing this, in 1977, the federal government changed the funding model by passing the *Federal-Provincial Fiscal Arrangements and Established Programs Financing Act* (known as EPF). EPF replaced the federal transfers that had existed for HIDS, the *Medical Care Act*, and for a third cost-shared program that had helped the provinces to fund postsecondary education (which also fell under provincial jurisdiction) with a new transfer payment. Rather than cost-share spending only for the activities specified by these older transfer payment models, EPF computed an entitlement for each province based on its population. In effect, the new formula assumed a certain level of need to deliver these services in each jurisdiction, albeit one that did not necessarily take into account differences in need that might be based on such issues as whether the jurisdiction had to serve rural or remote communities or even differences in the health costs for different age groups. (Subsequent formulas did incorporate various modifications that took such factors into account in different ways.) The formula also moved from one based only on cash transfers; instead, some of the payment was now in the form of tax points (whereby the federal government lowered its tax rates and allowed the provincial or territorial governments to occupy the vacated tax room). Only the residual difference between the provincial entitlement and the amount deemed to have been yielded from the tax points would be given in cash. The major change represented by EPF was that these federal transfers were now unconditional and went directly into provincial budgets. In theory, this freed the provinces to deliver these services in the manner they saw best, including shifting how, and by whom, they were delivered.

Not surprisingly, debates over the size of the transfer and the formula to be used have been (and remain) a perennial feature of Canadian politics. Although the per capita entitlement was supposed to increase each year at the rate of inflation, in the 1990s, economic difficulties led the federal government to unilaterally alter the formula, eventually removing all inflation adjustment for several years. One consequence was the erosion of the cash contribution. Since the imputed yield from the tax points would continue to increase with inflation, the residual difference that constituted the cash transfer kept shrinking. When analysts projected the trends, they realized that the cash transfer might soon disappear; this was due to happen first in Quebec, whose formula had included a heavier reliance on tax points (and hence even less residual cash). To preserve federal cash transfers (and federal ability to influence provincial policy), in 1996 EPF was accordingly combined with the 1966 Canada Assistance Plan, another federal transfer to the provinces which had helped pay the costs for certain non-universal social programs; the new transfer was renamed the Canada Health and Social Transfer (CHST). Federal-provincial discussions over how much money should be transferred and what it should be spent on continued. In 2000 the federal government agreed to provide an additional $23.4 billion to the provinces, of which some was earmarked for early childhood development, purchasing necessary diagnostic and treatment equipment, reforming primary care, and helping Canada Health Infoway adopt information technologies. Building on this, another First Ministers' Accord on Health Care Renewal, announced in February 2003, provided for an increase of $36.8 billion over the next five-year period, including some money purportedly targeted for primary health care, home care, catastrophic drug coverage, and new diagnostic equipment.[7]

In 2004 the CHST was split into two transfers; these were renamed the CHT and the CST.

Debates over health care programs continued. Proposed policies varied with different federal governments, which took different views about the extent to which they wanted to be involved with activities that legally fell under provincial or territorial jurisdiction. At the same time, following several meetings of the federal and provincial governments, the 2004 First Ministers' Accord on Health Care Renewal (commonly called the Health Accord, or the Ten-Year Deal), had been announced. The Health Accord again increased federal funding, provided some stability as to the amount of the transfer, and suggested some general future priorities (particularly around wait times, home care, prescription drugs, and team-based primary care), albeit with few mechanisms incorporated for enforcing these priorities. The Health Accord was sold as a major policy change. Under it, federal transfers increased by 6% per year. However, this agreement expired in 2014 and was not renewed by the Harper government. The federal government also refused to meet with the provinces to negotiate a new agreement; instead, it unilaterally announced that transfers would continue to increase by 6% per year until 2016–17 and would then be tied to the rate of economic growth and inflation (but would not fall below a 3% annual increase). It also made some modifications to the funding formula, including announcing a proposed cut to the CHT (which was to begin in 2017) and the elimination of the equalization portion of the CHT as of 2014. In 2015 when the Harper government was replaced by the Liberal government led by Justin Trudeau, the new government announced its intention to renew the Accord, but the precise formula (and conditions to be applied) was still under negotiation at the time of writing. The federal government's offer in December 2016 would have fixed the rate of annual increase over the next five years at 3.5% but offered an additional $11.5 billion over 10 years targeted at mental health and home care. At the time of writing, the provinces have rejected this as insufficient, but all the territories and provinces have subsequently agreed to bilateral deals. Negotiations continue.

As noted above, one immediate effect of introducing EPF in 1977 was that there were no longer any clear conditions that had to be met by the provincial insurance programs for physician and hospital care, since, as opposed to being tied to specific activities, the federal transfers now went directly into provincial general revenues. Indeed, it could be argued that there was no longer a federal transfer for health. That has not stopped the federal and provincial governments from battling about what proportion of health care is paid for by each level of government. There is considerable scope for creative accounting, both in terms of what will be included in the numerator and what will be considered in the denominator. Should the numerator include cash transfers only, or also include the estimated value of the tax points? Should the denominator include all health care costs or only the doctor and hospital costs that had been included under HIDS and the *Medical Care Act*? Depending on the choices, federal contributions will look larger or smaller. This dispute was reflected in the 2016 negotiations about the new transfers, where the provinces argued that the offer from Ottawa would have reduced the federal share of health spending from 23% to closer to 20% and argued instead for increasing it to 25%. Others might argue that these numbers have little meaning without clarifying what is being included in the numerator and the denominator.

Another immediate effect of EPF, however, was that some provinces began moving towards introducing user fees for services that formerly had been fully insured; such fees (which may include co-payments and deductibles) are often called *extra billing*. Some also argued that the move away from targeted funding made it easier for provinces to divert funds from health care to other purposes without losing federal transfers. This created an immediate outcry. In 1979 the federal government responded by asking Justice Hall to conduct a follow-up inquiry. What is sometimes called the second Hall Report was released the next year; although it was unwilling to conclude that federal health dollars had been diverted, it was strongly against allowing such extra billing. The federal government reacted by introducing and passing (again with all-party approval) the 1984 *Canada Health Act*, which attached some terms and conditions that provincial insurance plans would have to meet to continue to receive full federal funding under EPF. The same rules have continued to apply to the federal transfers under the programs that replaced EPF (primarily the CHT, since no similar rules were ever implemented for the social programs covered by the CST).

The Canada Health Act

The *Canada Health Act* (CHA) defines the terms and conditions that must be met by provincial (and, by extension, territorial) insurance plans to qualify for a full cash contribution from the federal government.[8] The CHA includes the following five conditions, which closely resemble those that had been attached to the older HIDS and *Medical Care Acts*:

1. *Public administration*: To meet the public administration requirement, the provincial insurance plan must be administered and operated on a non-profit basis by a public authority, designated by the province. This public authority can, with conditions, designate an agency to receive payments to the provincial health care insurance plan or to carry out on its behalf responsibilities in connection with receipt or payment of accounts for insured health services. The public administration requirement has sometimes been misinterpreted; it says nothing about how health care itself should be delivered and deals only with management of the insurance plan.
2. *Comprehensiveness*: The comprehensiveness condition requires the provincial plan to insure all "insured health services" that are provided to "insured persons" by hospitals and doctors, and

where the law of the province so permits, similar or additional services of other health care practitioners. An insured person is defined as a resident of that province or territory, more specifically, as "a person lawfully entitled to be or to remain in Canada who makes his home and is ordinarily present in the province, but does not include a tourist, a transient or a visitor to the province." The waiting period before someone is considered a resident cannot exceed three months. However, most of the provinces and territories also require that residents be physically present for at least 183 days per year, which is sometimes problematic for snowbirds trying to winter in Florida while retaining their Canadian health insurance. The CHA's definition of insured services will be discussed following the description of the CHA conditions.

3. *Universality*: The universality condition states that the plan must cover all "insured health services" for all "insured persons" in that province under "uniform terms and conditions."

4. *Portability*: Because the plans are set up on a provincial and territorial basis, the portability requirement specifies the rules governing what happens when someone who is an insured person in one province (or territory) needs care while outside that jurisdiction. As noted above, the definition of insured persons specifies that the waiting period before a new resident in that province or territory is eligible for insured health services cannot exceed three months. The CHA also includes some (limited) requirements for coverage when insured residents are temporarily out of the province. For care provided in another province or territory within Canada, it specifies that payment will be at the rate that is approved by the plan of the province in which the services are provided, although provinces are able to negotiate alternative arrangements if they want to do so. For care provided outside Canada, however, provinces must pay only the amount that they would have paid for a similar service provided within their province. For elective procedures, prior approval may also be required. This means that individuals travelling to jurisdictions where care is likely to be costlier (e.g., the United States) are strongly advised to have additional private travel health insurance.

The portability condition also specifies what happens when residents move from one province to another. If provinces choose to impose a minimum waiting period (which, as noted above, can be up to three months), the costs of any medically necessary care the people receive will remain the responsibility of the sending province for that period; this enables people to visit other parts of the country for a short time without imposing costs on the location they are visiting (e.g., if someone from Nova Scotia takes a trip to Banff and has a skiing accident, Alberta will not have to pay for the treatment). After the three-month waiting period, the person is deemed to have moved from one province to another (although the person may have to so inform the respective provincial health plans), and the receiving province will then assume responsibility for the costs of insured services.

These portability provisions have caused problems for immigrants arriving from outside Canada; since they do not have a sending province, they would not have to be publicly covered for their first three months in Canada, although provinces have varied in the extent to which they actually require immigrants to wait. In addition, because the universality condition deals only with legal residents of Canada, visitors (including foreign students) are not eligible for coverage and need to have private insurance. To minimize problems of people moving across provincial boundaries to gain access to services that may not be covered in the sending province, the sending provincial insurance plans also have the right to require that prior permission be obtained before paying for "elective insured services" out of the province. Emergency services, however, must be covered for insured persons.

The portability clause not only results in additional bureaucratic requirements for the provinces, particularly since what is covered can vary across provincial lines, but also raises coverage issues when people live in multiple provinces at the same time. For example, if students from Nova Scotia choose to go to school at the University of Toronto in Ontario, it is not always clear where they officially reside and hence who would be responsible for providing their health insurance. Indeed, similar issues have arisen for Canadian senators. As one highly publicized example, Senator Mike Duffy was appointed as a representative from Prince Edward Island, but he had been living in Ottawa and receiving most of his health care services from Ontario. Indeed, at the time of his appointment to the Senate, he held an Ontario Health Insurance Plan (OHIP) card, meaning that Ontario was paying for his medical care. The question arose as to whether having qualified for an OHIP card meant that he had violated the requirement to be a resident of PEI. At the time of writing, the issue of defining what province someone is a resident of had not been fully resolved.

5. *Accessibility*: The accessibility condition requires that the provincial plans provide insured health services to insured persons on uniform terms and conditions. These insured services must be reasonably accessible to all insured persons; direct or indirect impediments (including user charges) that would affect the ability of insured persons to receive insured services are explicitly prohibited. This condition also requires that the provincial plans must provide "reasonable compensation" to health care practitioners for all insured health services they provide; the amount to be paid will usually be determined through negotiations between the province and the provincial organization representing the medical practitioners. Disputes are to be settled through conciliation or binding arbitration. Similarly, the provincial plan must provide reasonable payment to hospitals to cover the cost of insured health services provided to insured persons. Determining what is seen to be reasonable is also an ongoing issue, particularly as provincial governments argue with their doctors and hospitals about how much money they will receive.

The CHA specifies that if a provincial health care plan does not meet the above stated criteria it will be subject to reduced or complete withholding of cash contributions or any amounts payable to them by Canada. As defined in the Act, these criteria thus prohibit extra billing or user fees for insured services; however, charging fees for services not meeting the definition of insured services (including accommodation and meals for those people in chronic care facilities) is permitted and will not incur fiscal penalties. There is also a requirement to provide the federal health minister with the information set out in the regulations on a yearly basis and for the provincial and territorial health plans to give recognition for the contributions and payments made by the federal government under this Act in any public documents, advertising, or promotional material relating to insured health services and extended health care services in the province. As required by the CHA, every fiscal year, Health Canada produces and posts a report on the extent to which provincial and territorial health care insurance plans have satisfied the criteria and the conditions for payment under the Act.[9]

The question of defining what is meant by medical necessity is a perennial issue.[10] As noted above, the CHA deals with it by speaking of "insured services," which it has defined as follows:

Insured health services means hospital services, physician services and surgical-dental services provided to insured persons, but does not include any health services that a person is entitled to and eligible for under any other Act of Parliament or under any Act of the legislature of a province that relates to workers' or workmen's compensation.

Hospital services means any of the following services provided to inpatients or out-patients at a hospital, if the services are medically necessary for the purpose of maintaining health, preventing disease or diagnosing or treating an injury, illness or disability namely:
(a) accommodation and meals at the standard or public ward level and preferred accommodation if medically required,
(b) nursing service,
(c) laboratory, radiological and other diagnostic procedures, together with the necessary interpretations,
(d) drugs, biologicals and related preparations when administered in the hospital,
(e) use of operating room, case room and anaesthetic facilities, including necessary equipment and supplies,
(f) medical and surgical equipment and supplies,
(g) use of radiotherapy facilities,
(h) use of physiotherapy facilities, and

(i) services provided by persons who receive remuneration therefor from the hospital,

but does not include services that are excluded by the regulations.

Physician services means any medically required services rendered by medical practitioners.

Surgical-dental services means any medically or dentally required surgical-dental procedures performed by a dentist in a hospital, where a hospital is required for the proper performance of the procedures.[11]

In practice, almost no dental services meet this criteria; dental care is almost entirely privately financed in Canada.

These definitions demonstrate a clear effort to anticipate and plug loopholes. When people are hospitalized, it is not permitted to charge them for their meals or charge them rent for occupying a hospital room. Similarly, if someone needs a private room for medical reasons (e.g., risk of infection), they cannot be charged extra for that, although they can be charged an accommodation fee if they simply prefer not to have roommates. If a hospital-given test qualifies as an insured service, patients cannot be charged an additional payment for interpreting what it means. Neither can they be extra billed for the equipment or supplies needed to provide an insured surgical procedure performed in a hospital.

As would be expected given the historical emphasis on hospital and physician care, the CHA also makes an explicit distinction between insured services and "extended health care services" (which are defined as including such things as "(a) nursing home intermediate care service, (b) adult residential care service, (c) home care service, and (d) ambulatory health care service"). Unlike hospital and doctor services, these extended health care services are not subject to the CHA terms and conditions and accordingly do not have to be publicly paid for; those using them may have to pay some, or all, of the cost.[12]

As this description of Canadian health care clarifies, since 1984, the federal-provincial arrangements for health care in Canada have operated under two separate pieces of legislation. One (currently the CHT) sets out how much money provincial and territorial governments will receive in federal transfers, and the other (the CHA) specifies what, if any, conditions need to be met to receive the money. It is notable that, although funding for postsecondary education and social welfare programs (including social assistance, social services, early childhood development, and child care) were also incorporated into these federal transfer programs, few federal conditions were attached to funding for anything other than the physician and hospital insurance components (although they were prohibited from imposing residency requirements on social assistance programs). Indeed, there is still no equivalent of the CHA for these other programs.

The CHA terms and conditions continue to affect Canadian health policy in multiple ways. One of the key issues arises from the definition of insured services. Deciding what counts as "medically necessary" can be contentious, even if services are given by physicians or in hospitals. One example occurs when your employer requires you to get a note from your doctor if you take a sick day; providers can (and many do) charge the patient directly for these. Although most hospital and physician care remain fully covered, the CHA definition of insured services means that, once non-physician care shifts from hospitals, these services are no longer required to be publicly insured, even though they may still be viewed as medically necessary. This has been particularly problematic for a variety of services, including outpatient pharmaceuticals (since drugs for inpatients are included within the CHA definition), outpatient rehabilitation, primary care by non-physician providers, and home care. Provinces can extend such coverage but do not have to. As I note in subsequent chapters, one reform that analysts frequently suggest, although it has not yet been acted on, is to break this link to doctors and hospitals and insure medically required services regardless of where these are delivered or by which providers.

The definition of comprehensiveness under the CHA is a floor, not a ceiling. It does allow provinces to expand the definition of who can deliver insured services; it includes the provision "and where the law of the province so permits, similar or additional services rendered by other health care practitioners." However, this has rarely been done. (There are some exceptions; for example, some provinces have designated midwifery as an insured service). It is worth noting that if and when the provinces do expand the definition, those providers delivering insured services would have to work under the same rules as apply to physicians; for example, they would be publicly paid for the insured services they deliver but would not be able to extra-bill their patients.

Another long-term implication of the CHA rules is that the public administration requirement eliminated any role for private-for-profit insurance companies to manage the provincial or territorial single-payer insurance plans, although they could (and did) retain a role in covering services not included under the comprehensiveness definition.

Subsequent to the passage of the CHA, Canada's history of setting up committees to examine health care has persisted. In 2002, two separate reports were published. Again, Saskatchewan could be seen as leading the way. The Royal Commission on the Future of Health Care in Canada, led by Roy Romanow (who was the New Democratic Party premier of Saskatchewan from 1991 to 2001) was established by the federal Liberal government in 2001. It generated a report, as well as a series of background papers on key issues.[13] The Senate, under the leadership of Senator Michael Kirby, also held hearings and published a series of reports, culminating in a final report and recommendations.[14] (I prepared one of the background papers for the Romanow Commission[15] and testified before the Senate committee.) Both the Romanow and Kirby reports came up with some remarkably similar recommendations, some (but not all) of which have been dealt with by policymakers. Other reports and analyses abound. Chapters 7 and 8 will deal with some of the commonly suggested reform directions.

Another ongoing policy debate, which we will discuss briefly in Chapter 8, concerns the prohibition of private insurance and extra billing for those services falling under the "insured services" definition. There have been a number of court battles, largely centring on whether the provisions in section 7 of Canada's *Charter of Rights and Freedoms* protecting the "right to life, liberty and security of the person" means that people have a right to access health care within a reasonable time and hence should be able to pay privately for care. One highly publicized court battle, *Chaoulli v Quebec (AG)*[16] related to whether Quebec's legislation prohibiting private medical insurance for publicly insured health care services was a violation of the Quebec

Charter of Human Rights. The plaintiff was a patient who had to wait for hip replacement surgery; he and his physician (Dr Chaoulli) brought a court case to argue that the patient should be able to purchase private insurance to move to the front of the line. The Quebec courts dismissed the case, but in a split decision, the Supreme Court of Canada ruled that the legislation violated the Quebec charter (although they did not obtain a majority opinion that it violated the Canadian *Charter of Rights and Freedoms*). The decision was seen as requiring that the province had a duty to ensure that people obtained timely access to insured services, although not necessarily through purchasing private insurance. Another court case, not yet decided at the time of writing, resulted from a long-running dispute between Dr Brian Day, owner of a private for-profit clinic (Cambie Surgeries) and the British Columbia provincial insurer (the BC Medical Services Commission). British Columbia charged that Day's clinic had been illegally charging patients for health services that were included under the definition of insured services. Dr Day charged that these constraints are an illegal restriction of charter rights.

Organizing and Delivering Health Care in Canada

As noted above, while Canada uses public payment for some health care services, almost all these services are delivered by private providers. This can be confusing, particularly since Canada uses the term "public hospitals" to refer to private NFP institutions, even though these would not be classified as meeting the definition of public delivery. Many of these hospitals were founded by charitable groups, including religious orders. (Canada still has an extensive array of Roman Catholic hospitals.) A few "private hospitals" (most of which would fall into the for-profit delivery category) do exist, but not many; the regulations under which they are (or are not) allowed to operate are set by provincial and territorial governments, and hence vary across Canada.

The delineation of what counts as public or private delivery has become even more complex with the growth of regional health authorities.[17] These regional bodies, which were established in most Canadian provinces starting in the mid-1990s, constitute a compromise between centralizing activities at the provincial level and decentralizing them to local organizations. For example, the management of hospitals was often centralized from individual hospitals up to the regional authorities, which often involved dissolving individual hospital boards in favour of a regional management structure. However, responsibility for allocating budgets within a region was frequently decentralized from the province down to the regional body. Depending on the province, these health regions have responsibilities for various mixtures of planning, managing, and funding combinations of services for their defined geographical areas. Every province has given them responsibility for hospitals, and (at the time of writing) none have given them responsibility for physician services (although Ontario has announced its intention to do so, particularly for primary care). Responsibility for other services varies; some provinces have given the regions responsibility for such services as community care, LTC, or public health, while others have kept them at the provincial level or left them within other ministries. Using the public-private model, these regional health authorities would fall into the quasi-public classification, since they are nominally independent yet heavily regulated by the province.

Alberta has moved the farthest towards centralization. It first eliminated most hospital boards and placed most responsibility for governing them with its health regions. It then eliminated the regional structures in 2009 and moved much of the responsibility for planning and funding the province's hospitals and selected other services to a centralized provincial agency, Alberta Health Services, which reported directly to the provincial minister of health and wellness. Alberta has implemented a series of zones and advisory councils within Alberta Health Services, but in effect its current model represents Canada's closest equivalent of an UK-style public delivery model, with most hospital employees working for the province. In general, most provinces started with a relatively large number of regions in an effort to look like they were still being responsive to local situations, but over time have been consolidating them and reducing the number, while still trying to maintain mechanisms that can ascertain and respect local needs. As another example, Saskatchewan started with 32 health districts in 1992, consolidated these into 12 health regions in 2002, and in January 2017 announced its decision to consolidate them into a single provincial health authority, arguing that this would reduce administrative costs.

Ontario was among the last provinces to bring in regional models, and its approach is the least centralized in Canada. In 2006 it set up 14 Local Health Integration Networks (LHINs) as regional, NFP corporations, but explicitly prohibited them from providing health services directly. LHINs are instead responsible for working with local health providers and community members to best determine the health service priorities of their geographic regions; their mandate speaks of planning, integrating and funding such "local health services" as hospitals, community support services, LTC, mental health and addictions services, and community health centres.[18] The Ontario Ministry of Health and Long-Term Care retained a stewardship role and overall responsibility for such higher level roles as establishing strategic direction and provincial priorities for the health system and developing legislation, regulations, standards, policies, and directives to support those strategic directions.[19] Unlike the situation in the rest of the country, the local hospitals and other agencies retained their own boards of directors, although most of their provincial funding now flows through the LHINs rather than coming directly from the province. The LHINs have accordingly been seen by some as an added level of bureaucracy. Ontario has been moving to align other health-related services along the same boundaries as the LHINs (although these boundaries are somewhat arbitrary and often do not match how people actually travel to receive services). More recently, Ontario has also been trying to align community services, primary care, and public health with LHIN boundaries. In 2016 the province announced that it planned to abolish the Community Care Access Centres (CCACs), the arm's-length agencies that are currently responsible for organizing and funding many community services, and to merge them with the LHINs.[20] At the time of writing, proposals had also been made to give the LHINs some responsibility for working with primary care and with the local public health units and to set up a series of sub-LHINs within the boundaries of each LHIN. This is likely to be complicated, in part because the current boundaries do not always align with how services are sought and received, and because public health is also partially funded by local governments, whose boundaries do not necessarily align with those of the LHINs. For example, different parts of the city of Toronto fall into five different LHINs, some of which also include parts of other neighbouring communities. In contrast, there is one Public Health Unit for all of Toronto. This would impose a significant coordination burden if public health was placed under the responsibility of LHINs.

There are also differences across provinces in how these financing and governance structures deal with specialized services that may serve multiple catchment areas. A clear example is a specialized pediatric hospital, such as Toronto's SickKids Hospital; it serves the province (and for some things, the entire country), rather than only the region where it happens to be located. British Columbia has an innovative approach; it has set up a region, the Provincial Health Services Authority, to handle specified highly specialized services that may serve the entire province, such as heart surgery, transplants, and cancer treatment. The Atlantic provinces of Prince Edward Island, Nova Scotia, and New Brunswick work together for some services; in the model they are using, most tertiary and quaternary care is delivered in teaching hospitals in Nova Scotia, with the other provinces helping pay the bills for the care their residents receive there.

Regionalization in Canada is a moving target, with each province making various modifications to how these regions are set up, how their boundaries are drawn, and what they are responsible for. In the final analysis, responsibility lies with the provincial and territorial governments, which can (and do) adapt to problems as they arise.

How Much Does It Cost?

Provincial and territorial governments provide data to a national body, the Canadian Institute for Health Information (CIHI). CIHI describes itself as follows on its website: "CIHI is an independent, not-for-profit organization that provides essential information on Canada's health system and the health of Canadians... Our stakeholders use our broad range of health databases, measurements and standards, together with our evidence-based reports and analyses, in their day-to-day decision-making. We protect the privacy of Canadians by ensuring the confidentiality, integrity and availability of our health care information."[21] CIHI collects, analyses, and disseminates a variety of databases on a variety of topics, including health expenditures, the public-private mix, and the supply of health providers. Most of these data are collected from provincial and territorial sources. CIHI also works closely with the OECD, and with the Commonwealth Fund, including helping them collect (and disseminate) Canadian data for international studies.

One key CIHI database tracks health expenditures. For 2015, for example, CIHI noted that total spending on health care in Canada was forecasted to be $219.1 billion, or approximately $6105 per capita. This was estimated as being 10.9% of Canada's gross domestic product (GDP). This represented a reduction in the share of the economy absorbed by health care; in 2009 and 2010, it had reached 11.6% of GDP but has been dropping since.[22] (Noted that the numbers CIHI reports do not always exactly match those reported by the OECD as shown in Table 5.1 in Chapter 5, owing to slight differences in how some of the variables are defined by different organizations for different purposes.)

CIHI divides health spending into the following "uses of funds": hospitals, other institutions, physicians, other professionals, drugs, capital, public health, administration, and other health spending. Not all these health expenditures represent clinical services; for example, the "other" category also captures health research. CIHI estimated that the largest share of health spending in Canada was for hospitals, but this was about 29.5% (down considerably from what it had been several decades ago); outpatient pharmaceuticals came second (15.7%), and physician services third (15.5%). One reason (although not the only one) for this high share of spending going to pharmaceuticals has been a shift from hospital care to outpatient care, since pharmaceuticals delivered within a hospital would be categorized as hospital expenditures, whereas the same products given to the same patients on an outpatient basis would be classified under the drugs budget line.

About 70% of Canadian health care spending comes from public sources, and the remaining 30% from private sources. This public share is relatively low compared to other countries with universal public insurance. Although this ratio has remained constant for many years, the share of public spending by subsector varies. This reflects the CHA requirements discussed earlier that publicly funded provincial insurance plans must pay for all medically necessary care given in hospitals or by physicians. For 2015 CIHI estimated that the public share was 98.7% of the physicians category and 90.4% of hospitals. (This is not 100% because some things like capital costs of building new hospitals do not fall under the definition of insured services and are often paid by private donors rather than through public payers.) The public share of other institutions (which includes some LTC facilities) was 70.3%. In contrast, the public share was 36.6% of the drugs category (although this only encompasses outpatient drugs, since as noted above, inpatient drugs are included in hospital budgets and hence captured by the hospitals category; it also includes non-prescription drugs that are not usually covered by either public or private insurers). The public share of other professionals was only 8.8%; this basically captured those non-physician professionals who delivered care outside of hospitals, often on a FFS basis, since those delivering services in other sectors (such as hospitals) would have been counted under the budget lines for those institutions. Because provincial and territorial governments are responsible for running the insurance plans for hospital and physician care, health spending accounted for about 40% of provincial budgets, although this varied somewhat by province, and also reflected what was paid for from provincial budgets, as opposed to being downloaded to local governments. This again requires us to recognize that ratios have numerators and denominators; for example, if social services or education was moved from being the responsibility of the province to being paid for by local governments, these costs would no longer be in the denominator.

Under those circumstances, the same health spending would then constitute a larger proportion of the provincial budget.

The public-private mix in payment means that there can be considerable variability in coverage, depending on where you live, how old you are, what conditions you have, what care you need, where it is delivered and by which category of provider, and what private insurance coverage you have. Prescription drugs are a particular issue. To add to the complexity, the federal government, through various programs, does provide drug benefits to some designated groups (specifically, First Nations and Inuit, the RCMP, the Canadian Forces, veterans, federal inmates, and refugee protection claimants); it has estimated that it spent $630 million in drug-related expenditures in 2014.[23] On the other side, about 10% of Canadians do not have any prescription drug coverage at all, while another 11% have very limited coverage and may have to pay a considerable amount out-of-pocket. One consequence of poor coverage is that people may not fill their prescriptions; a 2015 survey found that 14% of Canadians reported they (or a family member) hadn't filled a prescription in the past year because of cost, and another 9% didn't renew one or skipped doses for the same reason.[24] There is regional variation, but the research strongly suggests this is often penny wise pound foolish and can lead to worse health outcomes. Another possibility is that people may go to hospital so that they can receive necessary medications without being charged for them, even though they could be treated more economically in the community. There are similar issues around cost barriers to other valuable services that fall outside the hospital and doctor definitions, such as dental care, vision care, mental health, and rehabilitation. We will return to the issue of what should be insured in later chapters.

The Distribution of Health Expenditures

Averages are not always a particularly accurate way of describing things. After all, if you have one foot in a pail of boiling water and the other in a pail of ice water, on average, you are comfortable. Similarly, looking at average spending per capita is not always helpful.

With the aid of colleagues at the Manitoba Centre for Health Policy, Kenneth Lam and I examined health care expenditures for all residents of the province.[25] The Manitoba data set we analysed included all physician, hospital, and outpatient prescription drug use (paid from both public and private sources) for every resident of the province, carefully anonymized to ensure that no individual would be identifiable. Following ethics approval, we were able to compute the health expenditures for each member of the population. We used this data to sort the population based on their health expenditures that year from low to high. We then categorized them into 20 segments, each representing 5% of the population (which statisticians call a *vingtile*), except for the lowest spending group (with zero expenditures), which represented about 10% of the population. We also examined the top 1% separately, meaning that these people are included in both the top 5% and top 1% categories shown in Figure 4.1. If everyone spent the same amount of money for health care, then each 5% of the population would account for 5% of the health expenditures, and each bar in the bar graph would be the same height (with the exception of the bar for the top 1%, which would be at 1%). Figure 4.1 shows what we actually found for the fiscal year 2005–6, with each bar showing expenditures for physician services, hospital care, and drugs. Clearly, spending is highly skewed. The average spending was $2203.95 per capita, but 85% of the population fell below that amount, and the top 1% of spenders accounted for 35% of the expenditure. The lowest spending 50% of the population accounted for only 2.27% of health expenditures. Even breaking it down by subcategory, we found that 70% of the population incurred expenditures that fell below the mean for physicians and pharmaceuticals, while 90% fell below the mean expenditures for hospital care. Indeed, the bottom 50% of spenders did not use any hospital care at all.

We frequently hear that seniors are responsible for the high spending and are shown alarming projections about what will happen as the population ages. However, when we did the same analysis by age-sex groups, it was clear that although costs indeed differed by age group, the same heavily skewed pattern held; in every age-sex group, 80–90% spent less than the average for that group. One reason that

Figure 4.1 Distribution of Health Expenditures, Manitoba 2005–6

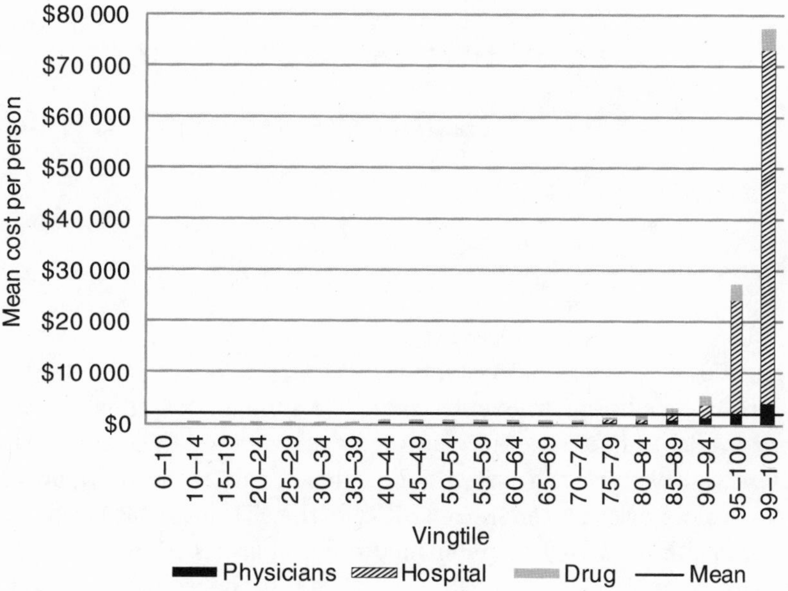

Population mean = $2203.95

seniors looked so expensive is that, as economist John Maynard Keynes famously said, "in the long run we are all dead." The oldest age groups thus incorporated the costs of end-of-life care, just as the youngest age groups also looked more expensive because they included the costs of being born in a hospital. The data pointed to two key policy options to contain costs and improve outcomes. The first is how we can keep the low spenders healthy. The second is how we can use resources more cost effectively for the high spenders. We will return to these points in Chapter 8 when we discuss the reform suggestions mentioned in the Introduction.

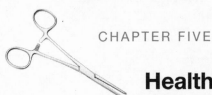

CHAPTER FIVE

Health Care in Canada: International Comparisons

Describing international systems is like trying to hit a moving target, since these systems frequently change. A number of online sources are available that describe various health systems. The European Observatory on Health Systems and Policies, part of the WHO, prints a series of health system reviews it calls the HiT, for Health Systems in Transition, as well as publishing other analyses of international health reforms.[1] The Commonwealth Fund describes and compares selected countries.[2] Canada's Evidence Network is an excellent source of information and includes a page with brief descriptions of particular countries and links to other sources.[3] These comparisons reveal similarities and differences in how health care systems are designed and managed internationally. As the WHO has noted, "a good health system delivers quality services to all people, when and where they need them. The exact configuration of services varies from country to country, but in all cases requires a robust financing mechanism; a well-trained and adequately paid workforce; reliable information on which to base decisions and policies; well-maintained facilities and logistics to deliver quality medicines and technologies."[4] Countries vary in the extent to which they meet these goals, as well as in the models they use to deliver health care to their population.

To compare Canada's performance, I have selected Germany, the United Kingdom, and the United States as examples of the other major approaches noted in Chapter 3. These countries were pioneers in implementing their models and are frequently used in international comparisons. However, it is important to recognize that no system is homogeneous and that even though the models we are briefly describing are the dominant models within these countries, closer examination would reveal some variability in how different populations and types of services are managed (e.g., Canada's model for financing dental care is not the same as the model it uses to finance hospital or physician services).

One of the first countries to introduce national health insurance was Germany. Medical historian Henry E. Sigerist traced its history in a classic essay.[5] As he noted, before the Industrial Revolution, the feudal lord was responsible for helping to care for those living on his estates, with charities being a back-up alternative. After the development of capitalism, however, people moved to cities, and the resulting burden on the charities became too great. Even in those early years, there was some limited coverage for different guilds of workers, including miners and sailors, but most of the population fell through the cracks. In 1883 Otto von Bismarck, then Chancellor of Germany and himself a feudal landowner, pioneered the use of what is now called *social health insurance*. Over the years, Germany passed a series of laws that extended the model. Social insurance is based on the premise that the public (acting collectively, often through government) has a responsibility to ensure that those who cannot afford care will get it but that others who can afford to should help to pay their own costs. The social insurance model is decentralized, using a series of competing insurance plans in the hopes that this will improve efficiency, although all of them are required to comply with government-set regulations (the nature of which vary across jurisdictions) to ensure that they provide basic, and standardized, levels of coverage, although individual plans can usually go beyond this. Social insurance models are accordingly funded by a combination of payments from employers and employees, plus government subsidies for the poor, although the cut-off for what is considered poor can vary considerably. Variants of social insurance models, often called the Bismarck model, are currently used in a number of countries, including Germany, France, Switzerland, the Netherlands, and Japan. In terms of the classifications in Table 3.1, this model is a mix of public and private (often quasi-public) financing, and private delivery. It differs from Canada's model in that there is not a single payer even for core services, although government will often regulate the competing plans. This social insurance model is similar to private retirement plans, where government may (to varying extents) regulate the sorts of private pensions that must be paid and how these plans must operate, while supplementing these with publicly funded plans for those with inadequate private coverage. In Table 5.1 we will use Germany as an example of the public or quasi-public financing-private delivery model.

England took a different path. Initially, the government paid for health insurance for some low-income workers, leaving the rest of the population to obtain coverage through private sources (both employer based and out-of-pocket). During World War II, the government felt it had greater obligations to help its people, particularly given the sacrifices they were making to help their country by fighting. Sir William Beveridge was asked to analyse the existing systems of social insurance that England was using. The model England ended up with, established in 1948, is named the National Health Service (NHS). Sometimes called a Beveridge system, the government not only paid for care but also delivered much of it. The precise model has been tweaked considerably over time. Since the United Kingdom consists of four jurisdictions, the NHS has separate units (which may operate somewhat differently) for England, Scotland, Wales, and Northern Ireland, although most international organizations reporting national statistics treat the United Kingdom as a single unit. In Beveridge models, most (although not necessarily all) hospitals are public – owned by the government, with most of the people providing care being civil servants. In effect, this model for hospitals resembles that for public schools; doctors, nurses, and other health care providers work in government-owned hospitals (which in the United Kingdom were known as *trusts*), usually as salaried employees. The major exception was primary care physicians, many of whom were self-employed private providers. However, government was the single payer for most care. Under the Thatcher government, the model changed somewhat in England to introduce an internal market, under which the Health

Authorities no longer ran the hospitals but instead commissioned care by setting up bodies to purchase it. At different times, responsibility for commissioning health services at the local level has been downloaded to various combinations of hospitals, primary care organizations, and regional authorities, with a varying role for the (still small) private sector. Modifications to the precise models continue (and often vary by region), but the NHS still largely follows a Beveridge model. Variants of this Beveridge model are found not only in the United Kingdom but also in other countries, including New Zealand and much of Scandinavia. In Table 5.1 we use the United Kingdom as an example of the public financing-public delivery model.

The United States took yet another path. Health care there is provided through multiple systems, but in most of them private financing and delivery have played a much larger role than they do in most other developed countries. Almost all delivery is private, with some exceptions (e.g., care for active and retired members of the military is often provided by publicly owned military or veterans hospitals). A series of competing insurance plans existed, with considerable variation in whom they would cover, for what, and at what price. Many of these insurance plans were private, but those over 65 and those of any age who had a few specified chronic diseases (including end-stage renal disease and certain disabilities) were insured by the publicly funded Medicare program (established in 1965 and expanded in 1972). The poor (with varying definitions, often depending on which state people lived in, of how low people's income had to be to qualify as being poor, and what would be covered) would be insured by the publicly funded Medicaid program. Medicare is a national program, whereas Medicaid is run by the individual states, and there is accordingly considerable variation in the types of coverage people receive, depending on where they live. Many people fell through the cracks and had no insurance at all. As would be predicted by insurance principles, those who had *pre-existing conditions* could be charged higher premiums or denied any coverage at all. It was estimated that, as of 2013, about 16% of the US population (about 44 million people) did not have any health insurance, usually because they could not afford it, while many others would be classified as *underinsured*, where they might still be left with high bills should they become ill. This contrasted with almost every other developed country, in which the full population was covered, albeit not necessarily under the same terms and conditions. The fail-safe was hospitals; according to US legislation (the *Emergency Medical and Treatment Labor Act*) passed in 1986, care could not be denied to people presenting to the emergency department at a "participating hospital" (defined as one receiving money from Medicare), even if they were unable to pay. If they were very ill, they would still have to be admitted and stabilized. Privately owned hospitals could still turn people away if they judged that it was not an emergency, but public hospitals (defined as hospitals owned by a level of government, usually state or local government, that receive public funding) could not turn them away if they needed care. This has translated into large differences in access to care, since public hospitals are not available in all locations, as well as a massive financial drain on these public hospitals, since they are often left with unpaid bills. It also does not stop the providers from still trying to collect their bills from these patients, including turning over their files to collection agencies. It has been estimated that health care costs were one of the major causes of individuals in the United States going bankrupt.[6]

In 2010 the United States implemented the *Affordable Care Act* (often called Obamacare); this retained the model of competing private insurance plans but regulated the market (including subsidizing some lower income people) and expanded the number of people with coverage. Obamacare still operates on a state rather than a national basis, with considerable variation in the extent to which various provisions have been adopted. Many state governments – usually those with Republican governors or legislatures – have refused to extend Medicaid coverage to the working poor. Obamacare accordingly did not solved the problem of non-coverage, although the number without insurance has fallen. Obamacare remains controversial, with the Republicans promising to repeal as much of the program as they can, while replacing it with an as yet undefined alternative. Given the distribution of health expenditures shown in Figure 4.1, however, as we will note in Chapter 8, allowing competitive models without the requirement that low-risk people still purchase insurance, which is what the current Republican plan proposes, is not likely to work very well. In Table 5.1, we will use the United States as an example of the private financing-private delivery model, recognizing that there is actually a mix of several models in that country.

Comparing Countries: How Does Canada Compare?

To see how Canada compares, we can examine the health statistics generated by various international organizations. This chapter briefly describes several frequently cited sources: the 2000 WHO ratings, the OECD comparative data, the Commonwealth Fund rankings, the (now defunct) Health Council of Canada, and Statistics Canada.

One widely cited set of rankings came from a 2000 WHO report entitled *Health Systems: Improving Performance*.[7] Its statistical appendix tried to rank all health systems; Canada ranked 30th in overall health system performance, while France ranked 1st and Italy 2nd. The United Kingdom was 18th. Although the United States ranked even lower, in 37th place, that wasn't sufficiently reassuring to Canadians. Closer analysis of the data found that the rating system the WHO was using had some notable flaws in the way it evaluated each country's performance. One problem arose from using ranks rather than scores; although there were indeed great differences between richer and poorer countries on many of these indicators, the scores for countries with similar levels of wealth were often quite close, meaning that tiny differences could lead to large differences in the rankings. Another problem was that the scoring system controlled for national levels of education, which artificially lowered the scores for countries (including Canada) with higher education levels.[8] Notably, the WHO has not tried to use this particular scoring system again, which does not prevent worried Canadians from continuing to bring it up when talking about health reform.

In Chapter 3 I briefly described the OECD and how it classified health care systems. As noted, its comparative health data is widely used. The OECD obtains its data directly from the governments of its member states and publishes them yearly, making them available online and through downloadable spreadsheets. It also works to ensure that countries are reporting data consistently, since otherwise seeming differences could be artefacts resulting from differences in how the data are defined and reported. The OECD 2016 data report[9] compares the following 35 OECD member countries, although which years each country reports data for varies: Australia, Austria, Belgium, Canada, Chile, Czech Republic, Denmark, Estonia, Finland, France, Germany, Greece, Hungary, Iceland, Ireland, Israel, Italy, Japan, Korea, Latvia, Luxembourg, Mexico, Netherlands, New Zealand, Norway, Poland, Portugal, Slovak Republic, Slovenia, Spain, Sweden, Switzerland, Turkey, United Kingdom, and United States. It also provides data for another nine partners who are not yet members but work with the OECD on some issues: Brazil, China, Colombia, Costa Rica, India, Indonesia, Lithuania, Russia, and South Africa. Recognizing that considerable variation exists among these countries and their health care systems, and that reasonable people can disagree in how similar each is to Canada, I used the 35-country data for the most recent year for which the OECD has published almost complete data at the time of writing to examine several metrics.

Table 5.1 represents an effort to extract and sort these data; for each of the variables selected, it reports the following:

- the metric and the "year or most recent year" that the OECD used to report the current data (which was used to generate Table 5.1),
- the OECD average (for as many of the 35 countries as it reported, which is usually all of them),
- the highest ranking country and its score,
- the lowest ranking country and its score,
- Canada's score and its rank, and
- the score and ranking for our three example countries of Germany, the United Kingdom, and the United States.

Note that on occasion this will lead to repeated data in Table 5.1 (e.g., if the United States ranked highest, I report that information in both the highest ranking country column and in the US column). On some metrics it is better to be high ranking (e.g., life expectancy), and

on others it is best to be low (e.g., spending). An additional complication is that "highest" or "lowest" may or may not translate into "best"
or "worst" in terms of performance; other factors clearly influence financial and health outcomes.

The first five rows we report in Table 5.1 relate to what is being
spent. The metric "health care expenditure as a % of GDP" indicates
the proportion of national wealth being spent for health care (recognizing that the OECD definition of health care spending deliberately
excludes certain costs, including many non-health care activities related to the determinants of health, but also such things as home care
services delivered by other than health care professionals, which it
instead classifies as social support services). The metric in the next
row translates this into money, reporting the health expenditure per
capita in *purchasing power parities* (PPPs), measured in US dollars.
The OECD defines PPPs as "the rates of currency conversion that
eliminate the differences in price levels between countries," which
enables us to see how much we are buying (defined in terms of the
volume of services). The example the OECD provides when defining
PPPs starts with determining how much it would cost to purchase a
litre of Coca-Cola in the United States and in France, and then aggre-
gating how much it would cost to purchase its defined basket of services in each countries. However, as the OECD warns,[10] these PPP
numbers should be used with caution to compare countries, since
they would not reflect efficiencies or inefficiencies resulting from differences in the prices actually being paid for these services, as opposed to the standardized price used for this metric. Accordingly,
PPPs per capita are commonly used to get a sense of the actual amount
of care being purchased (rather than the amount of money being
spent). The next row reports what proportion of the total health expenditure comes from public sources (which may include national,
sub-national, or local levels of government, depending on who is responsible for paying for what services in the different jurisdictions).
Confirming our classification of "compulsory health insurance
schemes" in such countries as Germany as quasi-public, it is notable
that the OECD has recently revised this metric to also include them in
the public expenditure category. The next metric reports what this

Table 5.1 Comparative OECD Health Data

Metric	OECD average	Highest country and score	Lowest country and score	Canada score and rank	Germany score and rank	UK score and rank	US score and rank
Health expenditure as % of GDP, 2015	9.0%	US 16.9%	Turkey 5.2%	10.1% #11	11.1% #4	9.8% #13	16.9% #1
Health expenditure per capita (US$PPP), 2015	$3814	US $9451	Mexico $1052	$4608 #12	$5267 #6	$4003 #17	$9451 #1
Public expenditure on health (% of total), 2015	72.9%	Norway 85.2%	US 49.4%	70.8% #22	85.0% #2	79.0% #12	49.4% #35
Public expenditure per capita (US$PPP). 2015	$2821	Luxembourg $6520	Mexico $541	$3262 #15	$4477 #5	$3163 #16	$4672 #4
Out-of-pocket expenditure per capita (US$PPP), 2014	$651	Switzerland $1815	Turkey $176	$644 #20	$664 #18	$586 #22	$1034 #2
Doctors per 1000 population, 2014	3.3	Greece 6.3	Turkey 1.8	2.6 #28	4.1 #5	2.8 #24	2.6 #28
Nurses per 1000 population, 2014	8.9	Switzerland 17.6	Turkey 1.9	9.8 #16	13.1 #6	8.2 #19	11.2 #11
Hospital beds per 1000 population, 2014	4.7	Japan 13.2	Mexico 1.6	2.7 #29	8.2 #3	2.7 #28	2.9 #26
Life expectancy at birth, females, 2014	83.3	Japan 86.8	Mexico 77.5	83.6 #19	83.6 #19	83.2 #24	81.2 #30

Table 5.1 Comparative OECD Health Data continued

Metric	OECD average	Highest country and score	Lowest country and score	Canada score and rank	Germany score and rank	UK score and rank	US score and rank
Life expectancy at birth, males, 2014	77.9	Iceland 81.3	Latvia 69.1	79.4 #14	78.7 #21	79.5 #12	76.4 #26
Infant mortality (deaths per 1000 live births), 2014	4.0	Mexico 12.5	Slovenia 1.8	4.8 #6	3.2 #20	3.9 #11	6.0 #4
Potential years of life lost, females ages 0–69, 2014	2288.8	Mexico 4600.9	Luxembourg 1562.6	2332.6 #12	2037.2 #20	2319.8 #13	3428.6 #2
Potential years of life lost, males ages 0–69, 2014	4409.2	Latvia 9051.1	Sweden 2892.3	3675.4 #20	3626.1 #21	3679.6 #19	5736.6 #7
Tobacco consumption %, 2014	19.3	Mexico 8.9	Chile 29.8	14.0 #29	20.9 #14	19.0 #20	12.9 #33

All data is for the indicated year or the nearest year for which the OECD had data.

public expenditure amounts to in US$PPP per capita. The next row reports how much per capita (in US$PPP) is being spent out of pocket, recognizing that this amount will vary considerably across the population, depending on different people's health needs. Note that the remaining health spending, which I do not specifically report in Table 5.1, would come from private insurance.

The next three rows give some information about inputs, giving the number of doctors, nurses, and hospital beds per 1000 population.

The next five rows give some information about results, showing the life expectancy at birth (in years) for females and males, infant mortality per 1000 live births, and potential years of life lost (PYLL) for males and females. PYLL is a controversial, albeit widely used, measure; it assumes that a normal life expectancy would be a fixed number of years (the OECD uses age 70), and then subtracts the age at which someone died (if they were between ages 0 and 69). The PYLL would thus be 50 if a person died at age 20, 5 if they died at age 65, and 0 if they died at age 75. Clearly, this is a debatable assumption, but PYLLs can be useful, with appropriate caveats, to compare outcomes across jurisdictions. A related measure often used by the WHO, not reported in this table, is called the disability-adjusted life year (DALY); it also attempts to measure the overall disease burden among a particular population by estimating how many healthy years were lost from being in a state of poor health or disability.

Finally, I include one metric related to health risks, giving the percentage of the adult population over age 15 who are daily smokers. (The OECD data set includes some other metrics dealing with health risks, such as obesity, but they have so many missing values that I did not include them in Table 5.1.)

This table does leave out many of the nuances, and the interested reader is referred to the original data, available at the OECD website.[11] Some minor differences may occur if similar data are retrieved from different sources. For example, the Canadian data are collected from the provinces and reported to the OECD by CIHI. However, CIHI often reports international comparisons data on its own website slightly differently than the OECD does. For example, for health expenditure per capita, the OECD reports "current expenditure per capita," which omits the costs of capital, whereas CIHI reports "total expenditure per capita," which includes it. For this analysis, I will use the data as reported by the OECD, since the differences are not that large and international comparisons are clearer if a common definition is used across jurisdictions.

Several things are evident from a closer examination of the data in the full OECD tables, although I do not include all of this information in Table 5.1. One is that the United States is a considerable outlier. One example is the metric for health expenditure as a percentage of GDP. The United States spent 16.9% while still leaving millions of its people without coverage. However, the country that ranked second, Switzerland, spent only 11.5% and basically covered everyone. Indeed, 10 of the 35 countries were bunched between 10% and 11.5%, meaning that small changes in the actual numbers could lead to considerable differences in where they ranked.

Another nuance is that ratios have numerators and denominators so that similar dollar amounts may represent varying proportions of national wealth. For example, Norway, which enjoyed an oil boom, was spending 8.9% of GDP on health care in 2013, ranking 18th. However, its spending per capita, in US$PPPs, was $5967, ranking it fourth. Because the economy was doing so well, this relatively high spending in $PPP terms still accounted for a relatively low proportion of the GDP. Conversely, if countries are not doing well economically, even relatively low expenditures may consume a high proportion of national wealth. Again, the United States was a massive outlier in its actual spending; in 2015, it spent $9451 PPP per capita, whereas the second-ranked spender, Luxembourg, spent $7765 PPP. Another nuance is that the PPP data largely reflect service volume, since the metric is computed by multiplying the volume of services delivered times the standardized price. If a country is more efficient in what it pays for these services, that would not be picked up by this metric.

A key message is that Canada is basically on the high end of being in the middle of the pack and looks quite similar to most of the European countries. Developing countries, such as Mexico and Turkey, are not yet doing as well economically, which affects their rankings. Drawing broader policy conclusions is possible, although this is risky without a clear understanding of the nuances of each health care system.

Other than the US model, most high-income OECD countries do provide universal coverage. One observation arising from closer examination of the full data set is that the countries employing a public financing model appear to enjoy better cost control than those dealing with competing payers in German-style social insurance models, although both models perform far better than the US-style model. It is also important to recognize that, to the extent this debate reflects underlying values about individual versus mutual responsibility, such data are largely irrelevant; if I do not care whether someone who cannot afford to purchase it will still receive care, the fact that it is more cost-effective to pool the costs and ensure everyone gets needed care would not matter to me. (This brings to mind the famous comment Dickens has Scrooge make in *A Christmas Carol* when asked to "make some slight provision for the poor and destitute." He asks "Are there no prisons? ... And the union workhouses ... Are they still in operation? ... Those who are badly off must go there." To the response, "Many can't go there; and many would rather die," he responds "If they would rather die they had better do it, and decrease the surplus population." Encouragingly, by the end of the story, he does change his mind.)

In terms of inputs, analysis of the comparative OECD data also reveals that the amount of variation differs across metrics. For example, Table 5.1 shows that as of 2014, on average, the OECD countries reported 4.7 hospital beds per capita, with Canada's average (2.7) being very close to that reported by the United States (2.9) and United Kingdom (2.7). In contrast, Germany had far more beds (8.2), implying that it delivers care differently with greater reliance on inpatient care. The number of doctors per 1000 population showed less variation; the average is 3.3, with Canada slightly below the average. Canada is also similar to international patterns (and slightly above the average) in its number of nurses per 1000 population.

Strikingly, relatively little variation occurs across these countries in ultimate health outcomes, at least as measured by life expectancy. Women have longer life expectancies than men, but the variation across countries is relatively small. Some might argue that differences of one or two years are significant; others might disagree. There is some variation in infant mortality, but that is affected by differences in what countries deem to be a live birth (particularly how deaths among very preterm infants are registered and reported), which can skew the findings. Canada can take some pride that it looks better than average on the PYLL metric, particularly for men; Canada has also had some success in persuading people not to smoke.

Another frequently cited source for international comparisons is the Commonwealth Fund, which regularly publishes a series of reports. They are based on surveys of the general public (age 18 or older) in 11 participating countries: Australia, Canada, France, Germany, Netherlands, New Zealand, Norway, Sweden, Switzerland, United Kingdom, and United States. They also survey physicians and other subgroups (including patients). In their general public surveys, they asked about 100 questions. These findings are subject to the same problems that any survey has (Is the sample size large enough? Who responds and who doesn't?) but do allow us to compare trends over time. In general, these Commonwealth Fund rankings place Canada near the bottom (usually 10th of the 11 countries they include).[12] Again, the United States usually ranks last. People can quibble with what the rankings capture, but they certainly point to areas that could be improved.

One of the most widely cited international comparisons on which Canada ranks quite poorly uses a series of metrics drawn from these Commonwealth Fund surveys (plus some OECD data). In the 2014 report, Canada ranked 10th of 11 countries, with the United States ranking last and the United Kingdom first. Breaking it down by category, Canada's ranking for quality care was 9th; this category was subdivided into effective care (Canada was 7th), safe care (10th), coordinated care (8th), and patient-centredness (8th). Canada ranked 9th on access, which was subdivided into cost-related access problems (5th) and timeliness of care (11th). The report also included other metrics of efficiency (Canada was 10th), equity (9th), and healthy lives (8th). The report gave Canada's expenditures per capita in $PPP as $4522.[13] This ranking has not changed much over time; Canada had ranked fourth of the five countries surveyed in 2004, was fifth of six in 2006 and 2007, and sixth of seven in 2010. The United States remained last.

While these reports point to obvious areas for improvement, it is important to recognize that the Commonwealth Fund scores are heavily reliant on how well the countries do with respect to such things as the flow of information through health records, rather than their health outcomes per se. For example, Canada scored quite low on such "effective care measures" as "Physicians reporting it is easy to print out a list of patients who are due or overdue for tests or preventive care" (23% saying yes in Canada, versus 88% in the United Kingdom). Other key areas of weakness related to waiting times or being able to see a doctor or nurse the same or next day.

The Health Council of Canada (established in 2003 and abolished in 2014), which participated as a partner in some of these surveys, also used its findings to compare results across the 10 provinces within Canada. In January 2014 it published its final report on the subject, which examined the results for 2013.[14] Several findings emerged.

First, Canadians were feeling better about their health care system. The survey asked people how well they thought the health care system was working. They were given three options: "1. On the whole, the system works pretty well and only minor changes are necessary to make it work better." "2 There are some good things in our health care system, but fundamental changes are needed to make it work better." or "3 Our health care system has so much wrong with it that we need to completely rebuild it." Whereas in 2004 only 22% had responded with the most positive response (only minor changes were needed), by 2013 this was up to 42%.

Second, and even more encouraging, Canadians responding to this survey were far more positive about the care they personally had received than about the system as a whole. Almost three-quarters (74% in 2013) rated their own care as very good or excellent. In addition, 61% of Canadians rated their own health as very good or excellent, which the Health Council noted placed them in the top 3 of the 11 countries surveyed. The Canadian respondents were also likely to report having a regular doctor or clinic where they could go for care. Depending on the province, only between 3% and 15% did not.

Results obtained by other surveys we examined were similar but not identical. For example, Statistics Canada estimated that in 2014, 14.9% of Canadians over age 12 did not have a regular medical doctor, with the highest rates being for those ages 20–34. Notably, this rate was considerably lower for those over age 65 (5.5% for males and 5% for females). The rates also differed considerably by province and territory, with five provinces or territories having rates below the national average (the lowest being New Brunswick at 6.1%, closely followed by Ontario at 7.5%), and six doing worse (including Quebec at 25.2% and all three Northern territories, with Nunavut at 82.5%); the remaining provinces were near the national average. However, almost half of those without regular doctors indicated that the reason they didn't have one is that they had not looked for one, and almost all of them reported having a usual place to go for care (often a walk-in clinic). These data also highlight the importance of nuance; Nunavut, for example, had so many people without a regular doctor largely because they relied on nurse practitioner–led clinics.[15]

On the other hand, access can still be a problem even for people with a regular doctor. Depending on the province, these survey results suggest that only between 31% and 46% could get a same-day or next-day appointment when they needed it. Not only did this place Canada at the bottom of the pack, but there had been no improvement since 2004. Many of those surveyed had indicated that when a problem arose that they thought could have been managed by their regular doctor if he or she had been available, they instead had to go to their local hospital emergency department. Most health policy analysts agree that this is not the best way to handle care. Not only is it usually more expensive to deal with non-emergency cases in hospitals, but it can also be both unpleasant and inefficient. When these cases went to emergency rooms, they would tend to be triaged into the low-importance category, meaning that these people often had long waits. (The Health Council report had noted that between 17% and 39% of those non-emergency cases going to the emergency departments had reported having to wait at least four hours before they were seen.) Another problem was that the information did not always flow back from the emergency department to their regular doctor, which might suggest the need to reform how the system is organized and how information flows across silos of care. We will return to those issues in Chapters 7 and 8.

Reassuringly, many international observers think that Canada is performing well.[16] Health outcomes appear better than those in the United States, although differences are not consistent.[17] That does not mean that there is not still room for improvement. We will return to some of these metrics when we examine some pressing issues in Chapter 7.

In the next chapter, we will turn to some ways of helping decide what is worth paying for. One set of tools is drawn from economics and talks about whether things are cost-effective and how to translate these findings into policy. Another looks at ethics and how they might help guide decision making. We will also look at who should make these decisions and what difference that may make.

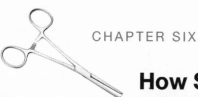

CHAPTER SIX

How Should We Decide What Is Worth Paying For?

Decisions about who should get what may occur at the micro-level (where decisions are made about how to treat a particular person), at the meso-level (where organizations decide how to manage care), and at the macro-level (when policymakers are deciding how much to allocate to health care as opposed to other needs, including cutting taxes, building and maintaining infrastructure, providing education, paying for national defence, and so on). As noted later in this chapter, who is involved in making these decisions will vary, which in turn may affect the weight given to different goals. Deciding what is the "right" thing to do is not always obvious, and sometimes there are varying degrees of right answers. One key question is what we're trying to accomplish. For instance, is the goal only to make my life better or to also take a broader view and look at the implications for others? In the final analysis, we cannot have everything, so we need some mechanisms for determining what we want to spend our money on (including how much we are willing to pay in taxes).

Economics can be helpful in looking at this.[1] One key idea is called *opportunity costs*, defined as the potential gains from other alternatives that you must forgo when you choose one alternative. In effect, you are asked to consider what else you might have done with those resources (where resources include but are not restricted to time and money). So, if you go out to dinner, you could not spend that money on a new pair of boots. Spending your money wisely would therefore require that you look at all of the things you might otherwise buy and make sure you select the option that would make you happiest. This sounds wonderful in theory, but in practice it can become somewhat overwhelming. Indeed, a full analysis would probably reveal that the opportunity costs of assessing all possible alternatives would make doing this a poor use of your time. In the example of going out to dinner with some friends, very few people will assess every restaurant they might go to rather than just picking the first one on which your group can agree. Economists do have some useful tools to help us evaluate our potential alternatives; they can analyse various alternatives, attach numbers to each, and allow us to rank the possibilities to pick the best ones. In health care, one key set of tools draws from economic analysis and can be applied to performing a *technology assessment* of proposed interventions. These tools are not always used, but in the view of many analysts (including me), they do offer considerable potential for improving the quality and effectiveness of health care.

Economic Analysis: What Does Cost-Effective Mean?

Economic analysis is a series of methods for comparing the costs and consequences of policy alternatives. A number of classic texts address how to perform economic analysis.[2] Although there are many complexities (including how to deal with uncertainty), these methods share a basic approach. First, they involve comparing alternatives. We cannot speak of something as being cost-effective without recognizing that we are only analysing whether it is more or less cost-effective than the alternatives to which it is being compared. Second, they require the ability to compute the costs and consequences of the alternatives. An economic analysis thus involves calculating the difference in costs between the pair of alternatives being compared (net costs) and dividing these by the difference in their outcomes (net effectiveness). We can then compute the incremental cost of obtaining an additional unit of benefit (e.g., many analyses of health care interventions look at how many dollars would be spent per year of life gained) or, if the consequences are negative, how much would be saved per year of life sacrificed. (In general, most economic analysis focuses only on potential gains.) However, doing this analysis is rarely simple. One set of questions is whose costs and consequences count; analyses can be done from various perspectives (commonly, patients, providers, payers, or society). Another set of issues relates to how these costs and consequences will be determined. The resulting family of economic analysis approaches has a wide variety of possibilities, including cost-minimization and cost-benefit, cost-effectiveness, and cost-utility analysis.

If consequences are identical for both alternatives, by definition, no incremental benefit exists. We can thus save some time, since it is not necessary to compute these consequences, given that the net incremental benefit will be zero. This allows us to use a *cost-minimization approach*, the simplest form of economic analysis, where we need only to compute the costs and then select the lowest cost alternative. One example might be decisions about where to purchase an item (or, similarly, which brand of an otherwise identical product to buy).

If consequences do differ, but they can all be expressed in monetary terms, then we can perform *cost-benefit analysis*, where we price out the costs and consequences and then look at the monetary return on the money invested. This is similar to calculating returns on investment, in which you pick the alternative giving you the highest return.

If consequences cannot be expressed in monetary terms but can be translated into a single common metric, we can do a *cost-effectiveness analysis* (CEA). For example, we can compute the number of life years gained, or the number of cases with a particular disease detected by a screening program, and can then compute the cost for each unit of benefit. This is sometimes expressed in terms of what are called *incremental cost-effectiveness ratios* (ICERs).

Cost-utility analysis is closely related to cost-effectiveness; it expresses consequences in terms of a common metric (such as life years gained) but then adjusts these for the 'quality' of those years. Commonly, quality is measured on a scale from 0 (worst) to 1 (best). For example, we might decide that living one year in perfect health would be rated as 1, death would be rated as 0, and living but being unable to get out of bed would have a rating somewhere in the middle. The resulting score we assign (usually on the 0 to 1 scale) is called the *utility* of that health state. We could then multiply the number of years to be spent in each health state by the quality of each and obtain the number of quality-adjusted life years (QALYs) gained by each alternative being compared. We can then use these data to help select the preferred alternative.

How to compute these quality ratings is highly controversial. One widely accepted method is called the *standard gamble*. It asks respondents to compare a sure thing (usually, living for a fixed period of time in a particular health state) against a gamble with two possible outcomes, usually specified as cure (valued at 1) or instant death (valued at 0). We then systematically vary the probabilities of these possible outcomes until the respondent is indifferent between the gamble and the health state being evaluated. For example, if people say that they would be equally willing to risk a 20% chance of death (and 80% chance of a cure), or to accept the sure thing of living for that fixed time in that health state, you can then say that the value attached to that health state would be 0.8. There is some controversy about whether certain states can be valued as being worse than death (i.e., have a negative utility). Using the standard gamble to compute utilities presents a number of potential problems. One is that it also confounds our attempt to measure the value of the health state by introducing the question of whether the outcome is certain or includes an element of risk and may thus also be measuring how willing you are to gamble (i.e., how much risk you are willing to accept). Another problem is that people are known to respond differently to outcomes if they are expressed as potential gains than if they are expressed as potential losses.[3] As one example, talking about a 20% risk of death may evoke different responses than talking about an 80% chance of living. That is why consent forms in hospitals often mention both.

A number of alternatives to the standard gamble are available if we want to measure the quality that will be assigned to a particular health state without having to consider people's attitudes towards risk. The *time trade-off* (TTO) asks respondents how many years in perfect health they would deem equivalent to a fixed time in that health state. For example, if they would see 15 years in perfect health as equivalent to 20 years living with the given health state, the utility attached to that health state would be 15/20, or 0.75. Other ways to measure quality attached to particular health states use different scales. Some may just ask respondents to directly value the health state (e.g., on a scale from 0 to 100); this number can then be translated into a utility score. Some break down the health state into different dimensions. Patients (or researchers) can use a number of scales to measure health status (e.g., the Quality of Well-Being; the EuroQol, and the Health Utilities Index) and compute a value for quality that can then be assigned to particular health outcomes. Another approach, willingness to pay (WTP), just asks people how much money they would be willing to pay to achieve a particular outcome and translates that into the utility score. This approach makes it easier to compare the value placed on health interventions with that placed on non-health interventions but also assumes that everything can be measured in monetary terms. These various approaches often generate different utility values, and there is currently no consensus on which is the best to use.

Some variability also exists in whose responses are used to compute utilities; these may come from the general public or from people who actually live with the condition being assessed. In general, those with more experience with the health condition tend to assign higher values to that health state than do the general population, which can be problematic if we are using these numbers to make resource allocation decisions for people living with that condition. Another contentious issue is whether assigning a lower value to life with a disability devalues the lives of persons who must live with such conditions and understandably believe that their lives are still valuable. On the other hand, without such quality adjustments, no value would be placed on interventions that may not improve their life expectancy but can greatly enhance their quality of life.

Another issue in deciding how to conduct economic analysis relates to how to treat costs and consequences that occur at a future time. The conventional approach is to discount these future consequences and assign lower values than for gains that would be immediately obtained. The choice of discount rate clearly can have an impact, particularly for outcomes occurring many years in the future. This is particularly consequential when dealing with disease prevention, since discounting can reduce the value placed on those long-term outcomes.

Translating Economic Analysis into Policy

After conducting an economic analysis (with whatever methods chosen), we can then take the results and try to translate these into policy recommendations. One possible approach, shown in Table 6.1, is to construct a three-by-three table that compares costs and benefits of the two alternatives being considered, which I have termed A and B. The columns compare the costs; A could cost more, the same, or less. The rows similarly compare the benefits, where again A could generate more, the same, or less benefits than B.[4]

Table 6.1 clarifies that these comparisons yield what we called *policy adoption zones*. Several are obvious choices. The cells classified as *don't adopt* indicate policy alternatives that should clearly be rejected, because they would involve paying more to receive the same or less benefit, or paying the same but achieving less benefit. Similarly, the cells classified as *adopt* would generate the same, or more benefit for less money, or the same benefit for less money. Indeed, we could argue that there would be no need to prioritize within the *adopt* zone, since all these would be classified as win-win situations. If the costs and benefits were the same, the choice would be a *toss-up* with no one caring except those selling the competing products. The *tough choice* zones come at the two corners, where we must decide how much more it is worth paying to gain some benefit, and, conversely, how much benefit one is willing to sacrifice to save how much money.

One of the most ethically and politically challenging parts of doing economic analysis thus involves deciding how much life is worth (which is often confounded with its closely related question of how much a particular treatment is worth). One example is pharmaceuticals. Increasingly, pharmaceutical companies are marketing products that offer minimal but non-zero benefits for a very high cost. One

Table 6.1 Adoption Zones: Comparing Options A and B

Benefits (A vs. B)	Costs (A vs. B)		
	More	Same	Less
More	tough choice	adopt	adopt
Same	don't adopt	toss-up	adopt
Less	don't adopt	don't adopt	tough choice

example was a drug being tested for one type of lung cancer.[5] A clinical trial found that it improved overall survival by an average of 1.2 months. Given the price the company was charging for the drug, it cost about US$80,000 to gain that extra time. Is that worth it? Patients and their families would probably say yes. Those paying the bills might or might not agree. If you adopt an opportunity-cost perspective, you might ask what else you could buy for that money and how many more people you might be able to help. This is a serious, and growing, policy dilemma. A 2016 newspaper article noted that the US Food and Drug Administration had approved 12 new cancer drugs in 2012, of which 11 were priced at more than $100,000 per patient per year. None of them involved a cure, only three even improved patient survival rates, and only one improved them by more than two months on average.[6] Payers, both public and private, asked whether this was a good use of their resources. A related problem is that if we agree that life is priceless, there is no constraint on the price that the manufacturers can charge. I will discuss who gets to make these decisions later in this chapter. I first focus on how this might be done.

One possible approach is to set a cut-off for how much you are willing to pay for a particular benefit. In the United Kingdom, what used to be called the National Institute for Clinical Excellence (NICE), which has subsequently been retitled the National Institute for Health and Care Excellence (still called NICE) used to say that any intervention that cost less than £20,000 per QALY would be considered cost-effective. If it cost between £20,000 and £30,000, NICE might approve it under some circumstances. If it cost more than that, it did not recommend funding it. After 2012, NICE modified its approach somewhat. One change was to extend the analysis to include other possible benefits (including potential benefits to the community, impact on vulnerable populations, and so on). Another change was to treat the estimates as guidelines only; some drugs are now being approved even though their ICERs are far higher than NICE's proposed cut-offs. Some scholars are arguing that the threshold should be even stricter, which would mean that expensive drugs would be less likely to be approved; as one example, University of York professor Karl Claxton suggested that the ceiling should be lowered to £13,000 per QALY.[7] In the best case analysis, of course, we could return to the adoption zones indicated in Table 6.1, and prioritize interventions that fall into the *adopt* zone of giving us better outcomes for less money. But this still leaves us with the dilemma of how to deal with those options falling into the *tough choice* cells.

One problem with trying to use economic analysis to make policy choices is that its language often generates heavy opposition. Economic analysis quickly morphs into the language of rationing – which has highly negative connotations – and then into "death panels."[8] Not surprisingly, most people reject the idea that any financial limits should be placed on doing things that might improve their health. Indeed, in the United States, the legislation implementing Obamacare contained explicit provisions that restricted the ability to use CEA in making treatment coverage decisions.[9]

Weighing Risks and Benefits

One possibility is to change the way the dialogue is framed. Instead of talking about cost-benefit, it might be better to talk about risk-benefit and about balancing the risks and benefits of various treatments.[10] An organization called Choosing Wisely Canada,[11] which will be further mentioned in Chapter 7, has noted that more is not always better. Its focus is currently on unnecessary tests and treatments, which it accurately notes may expose patients to harm without the potential for benefit; in the terms of Table 6.1, they clearly fall into the *don't adopt* zone. Eliminating such activities would seem the obvious choice if we got more benefit and spent less. But finding the dividing line between

Table 6.2 Test vs. Truth

	Truth: +	Truth: −	Total
Test: +	true positive	false positive	total testing positive
Test: −	false negative	true negative	total testing negative
Total	total with disease	total without disease	total

necessary and unnecessary interventions is not always that clear. In deciding whether to prescribe medications, we must consider what the side effects of a particular drug are and when the benefit is worth it. X-rays expose people to radiation; how likely must it be that someone has a particular condition before the benefit of detecting that condition outweighs the harm from the radiation exposure?

Epidemiologists have developed some tools for looking at diagnostic tests. Recognizing that some diagnoses are nuanced (e.g., opinions may differ about what the cut-off would be to define blood pressure as high), Table 6.2 presents how they would categorize the results of screening among a population who has undergone a particular test. The Truth columns look at how many actually have the particular condition being tested for (with Truth: + indicating the number that do, and Truth: − indicating the number that do not). The Test rows look at whether the test result suggests that we have that condition (with Test: + meaning that the test is positive, and Test: − meaning that it is negative). This table can be applied to multiple situations, including whether we have a disease, a particular genetic marker, sufficient knowledge of a subject, or anything else that we have a test for. Let us assume we are testing for breast cancer.

Assuming that we believe the test, four alternatives result. Those in the *true positive* cell have the condition (Truth: +), and the test so indicates (Test: +); we can then begin treatment if that is appropriate. Those in the *true negative* cell do not have breast cancer (Truth: −) and tested negative (Test: −); they can stop worrying, at least until they are due for their next test. The *false positives* do not have breast cancer (Truth: −), but the test indicated that they do (Test: +), while the *false negatives* do have cancer (Truth: +) that was missed by the test (Test: −). Assuming that effective treatments exist, two of these alternatives may thus result in harm; the false positives will receive treatment they did not need (and which may have harmful side effects), and the false negatives will not get the benefits from early detection.

How useful a test is thus depends on several things; we will focus on two that most analysts agree are extremely important.

First, how good is the test? This basically requires looking at the columns. Epidemiologists focus on two characteristics of a test. What is called *sensitivity* is the ability to correctly find disease; to compute sensitivity, we focus on the Truth: + column, and divide the number in the true positive cell by the total number who had the disease. What is called *specificity* is the ability to correctly rule out disease; to compute this, we focus on the Truth: − column and divide the number in the true negative cell by the total number without disease. Not surprisingly, tests vary in their performance. For example, estimates of the sensitivity of mammography for breast cancer vary from 75% to 90%, and estimates of its specificity range from 90% to 95%.

Second, we must recognize that the usefulness of a test also depends on another thing: how common the condition is in the population being tested (which epidemiologists refer to as *prevalence*). If a condition is rare, then most of those testing positive will still not have the condition. To analyse this, we use some examples presented in chapter 1 of *Case Studies in Canadian Health Policy and Management*.[12] As we will see, this requires looking at the rows.

To illustrate how these factors affect test performance, let us work through several examples. Clearly, for a test to be useful, sensitivity and specificity should be relatively high. For these examples, we will hold them constant and assume that our test has a sensitivity of 0.95 and a specificity of 0.95 (which means it would be much better performing than most tests). In each example, we will assume that we test 10,000 people. We will then vary the prevalence and focus on the rows to see how many of those testing positive actually have the disease and how many of those testing negative do not.

For the first example, we will assume that the condition is quite common. If the prevalence is 50%, 5000 people in the population we are testing will have that condition. Since the sensitivity is 0.95, our test will pick up 95% of the 5000 with the disease, meaning that we found 4750 cases and missed 250, who fall into the false negative category. We also correctly rule out disease in most people who do not have it, but since a specificity of 0.95 means that we will still erroneously place 5% of those without disease into the false positive category, we will have 250 false positives. They will have to get further testing or even treatment for a condition they do not have, which is suboptimal, but performance would still be deemed excellent, since most of those testing positive (4750 of 5000) indeed have the condition we were looking for.

But what happens if the condition we are testing for is less common? If prevalence is 5%, then 500 of our population of 10,000 have the condition. The sensitivity and specificity have not changed, so we pick up 475 of them, with 25 false negatives. But 5% of the remaining 9500 people without the condition will be false positives. Doing the math, 475 will be false positives, which means that fully half of those testing positive do not have the condition.

For rarer conditions, this becomes even more problematic. If prevalence is 0.2%, then only 20 people in our population of 10,000 will have the disease. We correctly detect 19 of them (with 1 false negative), but now have 499 false positives. Most of our positives do not have the condition. Epidemiologists refer to the resulting values as the *predictive value* of positive and negative tests. In our low prevalence example, the predictive value of a negative test is very high (even without testing, since we already know that 99.8% do not have the disease). However, the predictive value of a positive test was only 3.7%. At what point are we doing more harm than good?

These results highlight the dilemmas of focusing only on those in the *true positive* category, who are understandably relieved to have their condition detected early, particularly when early detection means they are likely to have better outcomes. A balanced decision, however, must also look at the consequences for those with false positive test results. How many healthy women should have a breast removed not to miss one case of breast cancer? Presumably, most healthy women would not be particularly happy to have received this unnecessary procedure. Indeed, this is one reason why recent recommendations have suggested reducing the use of screening mammograms for women without symptoms in age groups where prevalence is relatively low. A similar logic underlies suggestions to reduce the use of PSA tests for prostate cancer in lower risk populations. Note that this logic does not apply if people have symptoms (or genetic propensities) that suggest they might have a higher probability of having a particular condition; if you have symptoms, that usually means that you are in a higher prevalence group. As our previous examples have shown, a higher prevalence means that the test will have a higher predictive value and hence that there is a higher probability that the test results will be helpful. Indeed, under these circumstances, clinicians usually refer to such tests as being for diagnosis rather than screening.

Although this is not an example of screening, questions about how best to balance risks and benefits can be found in many clinical areas. Most treatments involve risks and benefits. Surgery can help or do harm. So can taking medications; as the "ask your doctor" commercials make clear, they do come with the risk of side effects, some of which can be very serious. Similar arguments could be made about how to organize care. One example is deciding when, and how, to regionalize treatment services. While this is usually seen as a question of trying to save money by not paying for services in rural-remote areas, there are procedures where outcomes are known to depend on performing a sufficient volume; going to an institution that does not do enough of them will thus, on average, yield poorer results. For such volume-dependent procedures, how advisable is it to encourage people to have them closer to home at a facility doing fewer of these procedures to avoid the inconveniences of longer travel time? The answer will obviously vary with the procedure.

Focusing on risk-benefit rather than cost-benefit gives the potential for some real win-win situations. The simplest is avoiding situations in which we spend more to achieve worse outcomes; having unnecessary surgery is a clear example. The logic of risk-benefit also allows us to identify win-win situations in which we can spend less to get better outcomes; one example is helping people control their blood pressure so they do not have a stroke. We may indeed need to return to the language of cost-benefit for the *tough choices* cells when we must decide how much we are willing to spend to gain how much improvement (and conversely, how much benefit we are willing to sacrifice to save how much money), but it is likely that there is enough low-hanging fruit in the *adopt* and *don't adopt* cells that we can defer some of these tough decisions.

Another way of expressing the effort to reconcile "the twin poles of ensuring access and controlling costs"[13] is to talk about *appropriateness*. Appropriateness will clearly depend on the patient and the proposed care; the term is basically defined as something that is expected to do more good than harm for that person. The WHO held a workshop on the topic in 2000; it wrote: "Appropriateness is a complex, fuzzy issue that defines care that is effective (based on valid evidence), efficient (cost-effective), and consistent with the ethical principles and preferences of relevant individuals, communities or society."[14] Properly defined, this clearly implies that one size will not fit all and that it is critical to examine the nuances of proposed treatments and how they are likely to affect the patient for whom they are proposed.

In the current environment, where we are often told to "be afraid, be very afraid," perhaps a recognition that treatments have risks as well as benefits may be more persuasive as a way of containing the cost curve than only focusing on costs. Ideally, we can find some interventions in the *adopt* zone that may even improve patient outcomes by not giving people therapies that are likely to leave them worse off.

Health Care Ethics

Although economic analysis can provide useful guidance for many policy questions, another important input involves incorporating ethical principles. The field of ethics is often rooted in philosophy, and there does not tend to be a single universally accepted approach. For example, ethicists may disagree about the extent to which the rightness or wrongness of an act depends on its consequences (which the philosophers call *consequentialism* or *utilitarianism*), or whether an act can be inherently good or bad, regardless of what happens (which they call *deontological*). However, some consensus exists on several basic principles.

One widely used approach to bioethics has identified four key principles, which it calls autonomy, beneficence, non-maleficence, and justice.[15] These are often called the Belmont principles after the 1979 Belmont Report, which first codified them. This approach recognizes that, although trade-offs among these goals are often inevitable, they are all goals that most of us would like to pursue. These ethical principles apply both to how a particular decision will be made, as well as (to a somewhat less extent) to our views about the resulting outcomes. Most ethicists agree that fair, open. and publicly defensible resource allocation procedures are critical.

The Belmont principle of *autonomy* says that we should respect people's ability to make their own decisions, as long as they are capable of doing so and as long as their choices do not hurt others. (In turn, this would imply that we need to ensure they have enough information to make a genuinely informed choice.) The principle of *beneficence* says that we should act in the best interests of others. One common example is that doctors are expected to act in the best interests of their patients; we would not expect them to recommend unnecessary surgery just so that they could collect the fees. In turn, this leads to questions about how, and who, should decide what is in the best interests of other people and what the limits of our respect for autonomy are when people want to make bad choices. *Non-maleficence* means not to do harm. This is not a new principle; *primum non nocere* ("first, do no harm") is one of the Hippocratic principles that underlie medical ethics. The principle of *justice* talks about the fair distribution of outcomes, recognizing that this might be examined in terms of various combinations of their costs, benefits, harms, and risks. Again, deciding what will be considered a fair distribution is not usually simple.

Putting this together, we may be faced with the limits of what is sometimes called *solidarity* – to what extent are we our brother's keeper? How much are we willing to pay to help others? This will clearly depend on what sorts of risks and harms we are talking about, what if anything we can do to alleviate them, the costs, and the extent to which action would infringe on personal freedom. Is it an acceptable violation of your autonomy if I try to stop you from driving your race car at high speed down a city street in front of an elementary school? Presumably yes, because you are endangering others. Can I forbid you from drinking sugary soft drinks? Presumably no, although I may be able to ensure that these products are properly labelled so that you know what you are consuming and to make sure that we have tried to educate you about the risks and benefits of drinking them. (In terms of insurance principles, however, I may be able to say that I am not willing to accept you into my risk pool or help pay any health care costs that may result from your poor dietary choices.)

Another influential approach in the ethics literature has been Aristotle's principle of distributive justice, which specifies that equals should be treated equally and those who are unequal should be treated unequally. When trying to use this principle to guide resource allocation, however, it becomes evident that defining what is meant by "equal" is not obvious. We could argue that unequal treatment is justified when resources are allocated based on morally relevant differences, but that just kicks the problem down the road. Which differences are morally relevant? Some are obvious – if someone does not need a particular service, or is very unlikely to benefit from it, we can clearly argue that they should not receive it. If I am not pregnant, I do not need the services of a midwife. For the most part, many would argue that such characteristics as gender, sexual orientation, religion, level of education or age, if unrelated to clinical need and ability to benefit, would not be classified as morally relevant differences, although others might disagree.

How much guidance do these ethical principles give us in deciding where to spend our money? Ethicists have suggested a number of approaches. For example, what does it mean to improve equity? As noted above, equity is defined as treating likes alike, but definitions of what "likes" mean are not always simple.[16] Stone illustrated some of the possibilities by using the example of how to divide a chocolate cake that someone brought to her policy class. The most obvious way is to give everyone an equal slice. But equity is not always the same as equality, particularly when there are morally relevant differences. In the chocolate cake example, what if someone is on a diet or has an allergy to an ingredient? What if someone already had a large meal and is not hungry? Stone suggests that three basic criteria underlie how we might approach the concept of equity when we decide to allocate resources; she calls these *recipients*, *items*, and *process*.

What Stone terms recipients asks who should count as a member of the group (in this case, who might be eligible to get a piece of the cake). In the case of dividing up health care, this criterion will often reflect what jurisdiction people live in or what insurance plan they belong to. Even once the group membership is determined, we may have to decide if there are relevant ways to subdivide that population so that we treat those in the same category equally but those in different categories unequally; this is sometimes called *rank-based distribution* and spoken of in terms of the concepts of *horizontal* and *vertical* equity. For example, workplace-based health insurance may give different benefits to full-time workers than to part-time workers. There may be different insurance plans for those in particular age groups (particularly children and seniors) or for those with certain illnesses. In the case of the chocolate cake, those coming to the class in person would be treated differently than those taking the course online.

Stone's second criterion for determining equity is termed "items" and asks about what is being distributed. Sometimes the item should be considered in isolation, but we might also look at it in a larger context (e.g., whether some people also had cake in their previous class), as well as consider the ability to benefit (which would exclude those with allergies and the dieters from being tempted by the offer of cake). In the case of health care, these types of considerations are clearly relevant to how we choose to allocate resources, since giving people treatments that would not benefit them would be neither helpful nor wise.

The third criterion is termed "process" and relates to how the decisions are made. A number of ethical frameworks focus only on such process questions and conclude that things are fair as long as we agree with the processes used to reach the decision. One influential model is called accountability for reasonableness (A4R). A4R sets out four conditions, which it terms relevance, publicity, appeals/revision, and enforcement. *Relevance* is defined in terms of the rationales for decisions, which should "rest on evidence, reasons, and principles that fair-minded parties can agree are relevant to deciding how to meet the diverse needs of a covered population under necessary resource constraints." *Publicity* requires that the decisions, and the rationales for them, be publicly accessible. (Others refer to a similar requirement as transparency; the transparency condition is satisfied if decisions are made in an open and accountable manner, often ensuring that there has been public participation.) The third condition requires that there should be a mechanism for appealing decisions and for revisiting them should additional, new evidence change our earlier judgments. Finally, there should be some mechanism for enforcing these decisions.[17] Bioethicists Gibson, Martin, and Singer have also suggested adding an additional condition, which they call "empowerment"; this focuses on attempting to minimize power differences in the decision-making context and optimizing effective opportunities for participation.[18] Indeed, increasing attention is being paid to involving patients and their families in making these decisions.

Resource allocation decisions, by definition, have winners and losers. The A4R approach hopes that the losers will be more likely to accept the decisions as long as the process has met these fairness criteria. This may not always be true. Political scientists often use a theory, called *scope of conflict* (associated with E.E. Schattschneider[19]), which emphasizes the importance of where, and by whom, decisions are made. In effect, scope of conflict theory makes sure that we recognize the importance of the institutions part of the 3I theory noted in the Introduction. It also suggests that changing which organizations are responsible for making decisions may in turn affect the results. As one example, the decision about whether to give a patient an expensive drug may differ if the choice is made by a hospital deciding how to spend its budget, by an insurer deciding what it will or will not cover, by a government deciding on what it will pay for, or by a court deciding what services people are entitled to. In turn, scope of conflict theory suggests that the losers from resource allocation decisions, rather than accepting the results, might want to revisit them and may seek to select the venue and the set of rules that would maximize their chance of winning.

Another approach used in ethics, the *precautionary principle*, focuses on outcomes; it argues that an obligation exists to protect populations against reasonably foreseeable threats, even under conditions of uncertainty.[20] This principle, which has become influential in environmental science, is heavily risk averse. As one example, it argues that where the potential costs of inaction are high, it is the failure to implement preventive measures that requires justification. In effect, the default position should be to act. Similarly, you should not approve a product for sale unless you are certain that it is safe. There are several versions of the precautionary principle, which differ in how likely the risk must be to warrant taking action, since reasonable people can differ in their definitions of what would count as "reasonably foreseeable." (Taken to extremes, the precautionary principle would lead to inertia; you should never cross the road, because you might be hit by a car.) This approach may also be encouraged by fear of lawsuits should these threats actually materialize.

One key issue is the extent to which the precautionary principle should be applied to public health interventions. Some have noted that, if poorly applied, use of this concept risks doing more harm than good.[21] The issue is not only the costs of acting, which can be considerable, but also the risks to future policy. If we implement preventive measures, we can risk looking like the boy who cried wolf—being the people who call for help when it's not needed who are then ignored when help is needed; ironically, to the extent that preventive measures actually prevent these adverse events from occurring, critics may well suggest that those interventions were not necessary because the sky did not fall. (The successful efforts to prevent computer systems from crashing when the year 2K arrived in 2000 are a classic example.) The resulting complacency can be harmful and risk future adverse events. One clear example is immunization policy; paradoxically, to the extent it has been successful, we have a generation of people who have never seen friends and family contract polio or become very ill with measles. As a result, they may become complacent and refuse immunization for themselves and their families. To the extent this erodes herd immunity, as noted in Chapter 1, success has the potential for increasing the risk of future outbreaks. The public health community often says that, if successful, public health is invisible (which does not help them when they are seeking budgets to keep making sure the population continues to be protected from infectious diseases). Determining where to draw the line depends on careful assessment of the costs and consequences of various alternative scenarios and on how much risk the public is willing to tolerate.

The ethics of resource allocation are frequently considered in relation to the concept of justice, and how to balance our desire (and the health care providers' duty to seek the best outcomes for their patients) against responsibility to others, including society as a whole. Some will argue that human life is priceless; others focus on the fact that resources are limited and on the opportunity costs of not being able to use those resources for other (potentially more valuable) things. As Calabresi and Bobbit have noted, sometimes there is no obvious best alternative.[22] Not surprisingly, there are a number of approaches that can be taken to deal with resource allocation, which are briefly summarized in the next section.

Allocating Resources

As previously noted, resource allocation involves the distribution of various resources (which can include money, goods and services, time, etc.) to various activities (which may include programs and individuals). Such allocation decisions may occur at the macro-level (e.g., what resources will be given to health care versus to other potential uses), the meso-level (e.g., what resources will be given to particular organizations and/or programs), or the micro-level (e.g., what resources will be given to specific people). Who makes these decisions may vary accordingly. For example, macro allocations of resources to various activities, including health care, education, roads, etc., are often made by governments at the national, provincial/territorial, or municipal level, and by other decision makers (e.g., those who run large charities). Meso allocations are made at the level of institutions;

for example, hospitals must decide how to allocate their resources across such programs as cancer treatment, cardiology, and dialysis. Micro allocations are made by providers and by payers at the level of the individual patient; this is sometimes referred to as *bedside rationing.*

A number of approaches to resource allocation have been suggested in the literature. One way to categorize them is by the methods that are used. *Markets* are designed to ensure that the resources go to those most willing to pay for them. This may be seen as maximizing efficiency if we assume that higher WTP means that a higher value was assigned to that resource by the potential recipient, although it also will reflect differences in his/her disposable income. *Political* methods use societally determined guidelines, which preferably will be applied impartially. *Lotteries* rely on chance. *Custom* continues business as usual.

Not surprisingly, these different approaches often lead to different policy recommendations. Underlying these disagreements are several related debates. One is ethical. If we follow the solidarity principle, we may seek to distribute benefits based on need and costs based on ability to pay. As noted in Chapter 3, however, the logic behind insurance models points us in a different direction; those likely to incur health costs are not attractive members of a risk pool, since they will be expensive, and other members will often try to avoid having to subsidize their bills.

Ethicists note that the lack of a comprehensive, widely accepted theory of justice often gives rise to unresolved issues in how best to ration scarce resources, particularly when there are not enough resources available to do everything. Daniels has discussed several of these.[23] What he termed the "fair chances versus best outcomes problem" asks what degree should producing the best outcome be favoured over giving every patient an opportunity to compete for those limited resources. The "priorities problem" asks how much priority we should give to treating the sickest or most disabled patients. The "aggregation problem" asks when we should allow an aggregation of modest benefits to larger numbers of people to outweigh more significant benefits to fewer people. The "democracy problem" asks when we must rely on a fair democratic process as the only way to determine what constitutes a fair rationing outcome.

A related principle, sometimes called the rule of rescue, says that we have a moral obligation to rescue identifiable individuals in immediate peril, regardless of the cost. The tension between cost-effectiveness and the rule of rescue can generate serious ethical and political difficulties for those faced with making resource allocation decisions. Some also suggest that the stress on identifiable individuals tends to devalue prevention; it is difficult to identify a specific person who did not catch an infectious disease because he or she was immunized, or who was not injured in an automobile accident because he or she was wearing a seatbelt. Not surprisingly, economists are usually uncomfortable with the rule of rescue, particularly to the extent that it ignores opportunity costs.

Who Should Decide?

Another key issue is who should make these decisions. Clearly, the participants will differ depending on whether decisions are being made at the micro-, meso-, or macro-level. Let us briefly return to the question of whether a patient should receive an expensive drug, and, if the answer is yes, who should pay for it. This involves confronting a series of sub-questions: Should we offer the drug at all? Should we offer it to this patient? Should someone other than the patient pay the bill?

Here, the 3I framework – ideas, institutions, and interests – that we noted in Chapter 1 can be helpful. If we begin with the sub-question of whether we should offer the drug at all, ideas are clearly important. For example, we would want to know whether the drug would be helpful to that patient. Since people may respond differently, we probably will have to express the answer as a probability rather than as a clear yes or no. In that case, we will have to judge whether we have a threshold for considering the probability high enough, and if so, what that threshold would be. In addition, how should we handle the possibility that it may have serious side effects that would do more harm than good? People may vary in their views about how likely (and large) a benefit must be, and what risks might be involved, to warrant offering it as an option. There are also likely to be differences in the priorities different people give to different policy goals. For example, although some might argue that the policy goal of autonomy means that people should be free to take any product they want, most would probably agree that the policy goal of security means that dangerous and ineffective products should not be offered to patients. Some might adopt a "buyer beware" philosophy and allow these goods to remain available even if useless or harmful. However, even among those placing a higher priority on autonomy than on security, most would probably agree that other people (usually via public or private insurers) should not be required to pay for such products.

The institutions involved in deciding the first sub-question – whether the drug can be sold at all – are largely regulatory; most countries have drug approval bodies that must judge whether a product is sufficiently safe, and sufficiently effective, to be approved for sale. In Canada, this is done at the federal level, and at the time of writing was the responsibility of the Health Products and Food Branch (HPFB) of Health Canada. An obvious trade-off occurs between giving people rapid access to medicines that might be helpful even if the evidence is incomplete and ensuring that the products being offered are safe; analysts differ about where the line should be drawn. (At the time of writing, Canada did tend to try to expedite access, which accordingly meant that it was approving more drugs that subsequently had to have serious safety warnings.[24]) In addition, a process does exist to allow physicians to prescribe drugs that have not yet been approved (the Special Access Program, also administered by the HPFB branch). Note that the regulatory process varies by type of product; for example, Canada and the United States tend not to regulate natural products as heavily as they do prescription drugs. However, these products can still place people at risk. As one example, a 2016 newspaper story noted that a teenager had purchased an "all-natural" weight loss product at a big-box store and nearly died of liver failure, which resulted from the "green tea extract" in the product.[25]

The second sub-question of whether we should offer it to this patient usually involves discussions between individual patients and their providers, and draws on clinical judgments and preferences, although clinicians may also suggest clinical guidelines for when treatments should or should not be prescribed.

Once we decide whether the product should be approved for use, we may consider the question of who should pay for it. As the third sub-question of whether someone other than the patient should pay the bill highlights, however, the decision to approve a drug does not necessarily mean that it should be publicly paid for.

Clearly, we are now dealing with a different set of ideas, institutions, and interests. In making these funding decisions, some of the key ideas will relate to our views about solidarity and the extent to which we should pay to help others. The institutions will also differ; decisions may be made within a particular hospital (which may have some autonomy to decide how to spend its hospital budget), by private insurance plans, or by a publicly funded plan. If someone sues, the authority to make these decisions may move to the courts. Policy analysts note that changing the institutions also implies changing the interests, since different stakeholders will have different roles in different decision-making structures. Another factor that is often influential is media coverage about a particular individual who wants to receive that drug. If that person (and the family) is sufficiently sympathetic to evoke public interest and support, payers may come under increased pressure to approve coverage, even if the evidence of benefit, or its value for money using economic analysis, is slim.

Who makes these decisions will thus vary by jurisdiction. One key set of institutions that affect these decisions in Canada was set up in 1989 by Canada's federal and provincial and territorial governments. The Canadian Coordinating Office for Health Technology Assessment – which has changed its name to the Canadian Agency for Drugs and Technology in Health (CADTH) – was given the mandate to perform health technology assessment and thereby assist the provinces and territories when they needed to make decisions about whether to pay for particular products. Although CADTH's recommendations are advisory, it is heavily involved in the earlier stages of these decisions, particularly in reviewing pharmaceutical products. The branches include the Common Drug Review, and the pan-Canadian Oncology Drug Review, as well as an ability to do Rapid Responses.[26] (It also offers FFS consultations to pharmaceutical companies about how best to present evidence to the review bodies.) A related set of decisions (which will be mentioned in Chapter 8) deals with what price will be paid, and whether there are institutions tasked with trying to set these prices.

The interests who will become involved in making these decisions will also vary. What we called the *concentrated interests* in Chapter 1 are most likely to try to be at the table; this will include the people who have illnesses that they think (or hope) would benefit from the drug, their families and others who care for them, their health care providers, the pharmaceutical companies (who would like to ensure that their products will be profitable), and those who pay the bills. The general public, in contrast, would be classified as *diffuse interests* – they have some interest (particularly if their taxes, or insurance premiums, have to cover the costs), but they also have many other things on their mind and are far less likely to devote much attention to this particular issue. An additional complexity is that some of those with the strongest interests may be too ill, or too busy dealing with their health problems, to be able to participate. One non-pharmaceutical example, which happened many years ago, was Ontario's efforts to analyse what home care services people wanted by holding a series of public consultations.[27] The people who attended these sessions told them that people needed help with ADL; they placed little emphasis on getting more specialized professional services in the community to deal with more complex clinical needs. To the government's surprise, that was not what they saw once the home care programs were introduced. They realized that neither those with severe problems nor their caregivers had come to these citizen meetings, probably because they were too ill or too busy caring for their sick family members. However, those people did constitute a large proportion of those being served once the home care programs had been put in place. The programs had to be revised accordingly to ensure that the care needs of those actually using the programs would be addressed.

The Role of the Patient

Another important factor that is receiving increasing attention is what is often termed *patient-centred care*. The US Institute of Medicine has defined it as "providing care that is respectful of and responsive to individual patient preferences, needs, and values, and ensuring that patient values guide all clinical decisions."[28] This has led to an increasing emphasis on patient engagement and patient empowerment as ways of ensuring that their views are heard, along with some confusion as to what this actually means.

For example, at the micro-level, there is dispute about whether patient empowerment implies that patients should receive whatever treatment they desire, regardless of professional views about how likely it is to be effective (or even if it is likely to do more harm than good). Are patients really customers who know best what they want? If so, what is the role of health care professionals? If you accept the view that patients should get what they want, what should providers do if they think that a patient is making a bad choice? If patients find suggestions online that their cancer might be cured by a naturopathic remedy, should the provider agree? To what extent does the injunction for providers to do no harm imply that inappropriate care should not be provided at all, regardless of who is paying for it? Particularly given the power and knowledge imbalance that often exists between physician and patient, to what extent does the physician have a fiduciary duty to promote the patient's best interest?

The extent of this ethical duty, which is fundamental to the physician's role in resource allocation, is also a matter of controversy. Some argue that physicians should do everything they believe might benefit a particular patient, without taking costs or other societal considerations into account. Others do not. An additional dilemma occurs when people are making decisions on behalf of others. This may include parents deciding what treatment their children should, or should not, receive and caregivers caring for adults who are not deemed competent decision makers (e.g., people with dementia). There have been a number of court cases where parents did not want their children to have to undergo chemotherapy, in the hope that less painful treatments might cure them. (All too often, the child died.) Another example occurred in 2012, when two Alberta parents decided to treat their 19-month old son with natural remedies. The boy died from meningitis; in 2016 a jury convicted the parents of failing to provide the necessities of life, accepting the Crown's argument that they had an obligation to follow a legal standard of care.[29]

One potentially useful distinction recognizes that treatment decision making is more complex than this all-or-nothing model. It also recognizes that patients may not want to be customers. My colleagues and I have postulated that making treatment decisions can be divided into two sets of tasks. What we call "problem solving" is preference-independent; it does not matter what you would like the diagnosis to be or your preferences about the likely effects of particular treatments – they are what they are. In contrast, what we call "decision making" does involve patient preferences, looking at such things as how people feel about particular outcomes and how much risk they are willing to take. If you ask how much I would care if I will no longer be able to hurl a fastball, the answer would clearly vary. If I were trying to make a living as a baseball pitcher, I would presumably care a lot. On the other hand, if I never played baseball, presumably this would not be a major factor in my decision making. We were able to classify peoples' preferred roles into one of three categories. "Autonomous" people wanted to be involved in both the problem-solving and decision-making tasks. "Passive" people wanted to hand both over to their health care provider. "Shared" people wanted to hand over the problem-solving tasks but to be informed and involved in the decision making. Our research found that almost no one wanted to take an autonomous role; those who did expressed a lack of trust in their doctor.[30] Most preferred a shared role in treatment decisions – they wanted their physician to do the problem solving but to inform them about the findings and their options, and to partner with them in doing the decision making tasks; this is often termed "shared decision making."[31] In turn, this requires that the information be clear and understandable, and that clinicians be effective in communicating with their patients. (The evidence is clear that effective communication improves quality of care.) One suggestion is that patients should not be treated as customers but as partners. Certainly, patient engagement is receiving increasing emphasis in many jurisdictions.

To sum up the topic of this chapter, how should we decide what is worth paying for? This is another example where we are dealing with trade-offs; there is no clear answer. Depending on the sort of issue and how care is organized and paid for, these decisions may happen in many institutions and involve many interests and many ideas. Some decisions are made by the individuals needing care and their families, others by those providing the services, those paying for them, and those setting rules and policies. As noted in Chapter 3, different ways of financing and delivering care contain different sets of incentives and may change who is making decisions and how much these decisions are allowed to vary across patients and providers. However, there would appear to be considerable scope for improving priority setting and avoiding alternatives that result in little (or no) value for money. Since so many decisions depend on the precise details of the individual needing care, implementing such changes will rarely be feasible as top-down rules; they will usually require working with clinicians, patients, and families to ensure that the resulting decisions are the best ones for that particular situation. Policymakers are increasingly attempting to make these decisions more evidence based, or at least evidence informed, but all recognize that this is rarely simple.

The next chapter will draw on the concepts referred to in this book to focus on several of the pressing issues affecting health policy in Canada.

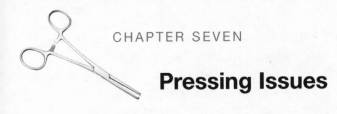

CHAPTER SEVEN

Pressing Issues

In this chapter, I will focus on a number of issues that affect our diagnosis of elements of Canadian health care that may need treatment. Reassuringly, there is considerable, although not complete, overlap between my diagnosis and those made by other experts on Canadian health policy. For example, a recent volume by Danielle Martin, which was published after this book was written and draws on her considerable clinical experience, seems to have made similar diagnoses.[1] The issues we will discuss here include equity, access to care (including wait times), quality and patient safety, accountability, and cost control. These may assist us in diagnosing what we think could be targets for policy change to improve health care in Canada. In Chapter 8, I will then address some of the reform suggestions noted in the Introduction of the book.

Equity

Health status varies. To the extent that these differences relate to the social determinants of health noted in Chapter 1, some of them might be avoidable with appropriate interventions. A number of organizations have called for paying more attention to how to reduce what they call inequities in health, many of which have been demonstrated to be strongly related to differences in income and education. For example, at the time of writing, considerable attention was being focused on Canada's First Nations and how to improve their health and living conditions, which are far worse than those of most other Canadians.

One key policy question is whether, and how, we want to reduce these inequalities, which can be seen both across and within nations. One key report was written by the World Health Organization (WHO).[2] In an extensive review, WHO called for three principles of action. The first principle was to improve daily living conditions, with a strong emphasis on early child development and education, improvements in living and working conditions, and the creation of conditions to allow people to flourish. The second principle was to "tackle the inequitable distribution of power, money, and resources" which involved the need for both governments and private organizations to modify how society is organized. The third principle was to better measure and understand the problem, and assess the impact of actions. WHO's extensive set of recommendations clearly reflected a social determinants of health viewpoint, with most of the recommended activities falling outside the realm of the health care system.

In that context, it is notable that much of the literature often assumes that equity (which we discussed in the previous chapter) is the same as equality, and that we should strive for equal outcomes. What this approach often fails to recognize is that we can achieve more equal outcomes not only by levelling up but also by levelling down. Let us compare two workers. One works for the public sector; she receives a guaranteed pension plan and a package of health benefits. The other works on short-term contracts in the private sector; her employer does not offer a pension plan or a benefit package. One view of equity would argue for taking away the benefits from the public employee so that both would be equally poor. The other would argue for extending these benefits to all. Politically, in many countries, it has been easier to mobilize resentment from the have-nots to level down than to mobilize support for increasing taxation levels or regulation to improve benefits and level up.

Another example can be seen when examining the success of policies aimed at improving the determinants of health. Consider anti-tobacco programs. Tobacco use is known to be a major contributor to a number of diseases, not only lung cancer but also cardiovascular and respiratory disease. It is also known that stopping smoking will reduce these problems. In theory, this is a win-win: people are healthier, and payers spend less on the costs of treating smoking-related illnesses. (It is worth noting that some health economists disagree; they have argued that tobacco use should be seen as cost saving, since, among other things, it kills people off quickly at about the age when they would otherwise have started to claim their pensions.[3]) In many developed countries, including Canada, these anti-tobacco programs have been highly successful. The rate of tobacco use has dropped. In the 1960s, it was estimated that about 50% of all Canadians smoked, whereas at the time of writing, the rate was estimated to have dropped to about 20%. Smoking has moved from being considered cool to being socially unacceptable among many people. Whereas in older movies, the stars all seemed to smoke, smoking tends now to be seen as a sign of ignorance and rebellion, which may be one reason why there has been a recent upsurge among the young.[4]

Paradoxically, much of this success in addressing the determinants of health has made equity worse. The better educated have been more likely to respond to the information about how to live a healthier life. Smoking is currently more common among certain sub-populations, particularly those with lower income and lower education.[5] Similar patterns can be shown with other determinants of health. The better educated usually eat healthier diets and are less likely to be obese. Although they may enjoy a nice glass of wine, they are less likely to abuse substances. Their health outcomes have improved more than those with less education. This leaves those adopting a simplistic approach to equity with a dilemma: are programs that improve overall health status, but improve it more among those of higher incomes, a good thing? Most of us would say yes; we are unlikely to want to level down and ensure everyone's health status is as bad as the least healthy members of the population. This in turn implies that a focus on equity alone may be inadequate. Instead, we may want to focus on *targeted improvement* and seeing how we could get better results among these vulnerable populations. In terms of the policy instruments we described in Chapter 1, this may imply an assortment of possibilities. In addition to using exhortation to make smoking seem less glamorous, we may want to use expenditure to incorporate tobacco prevention programs into primary care and other services, use taxation to increase the cost of tobacco products, use regulation to make cigarettes less available (particularly near schools), and change the packaging to incorporate clearer health warnings.

The recognition that we often face trade-offs among policy goals also plays an important role in clarifying why different policies are received differently. One clear example is the difference between our views about how to discourage people from drinking sugary soft drinks and how to discourage people from smoking. Both are clearly bad for our health. Yet in the case of soft drinks, we have been reluctant to intrude on people's autonomy and forbid people from drinking them. We may implement policies that require nutritional labelling (although having this information readily available is less common when one buys these drinks in restaurants or fast-food shops), because labels can be seen as giving people information to help them make better informed decisions that reflect their personal preferences, without restricting their freedom of choice. Placing higher taxes on less healthy products, however, usually evokes considerable opposition, and outright bans on such products are extremely uncommon unless the products can be shown to be overtly dangerous. In contrast, bans on public smoking are far more common. The usual rationale for such bans relates to *externalities*; because second hand smoke can harm others, respect for autonomy requires that we balance off the autonomy of the smoker against the autonomy of those standing or sitting near them. Much as we are not allowed to drink and drive, most societies have determined that we should not be allowed to increase the risk of cancer among the non-smokers who happen to be in the same bars, cars, trains or restaurants and have to breathe in our smoke, or among the children who share our household.

Various interpretations of what it means to strive for greater equity can affect our policies about resource distribution. For example, as noted in Chapter 6, people may give different answers as to the extent we should consider ability to benefit in deciding whether to pay for a treatment. Does equity mean that everyone with a particular condition has a right to particular therapies or that we should try to maximize the benefits to the full population? There is no one right answer (although, as I have argued in this book, there are likely to be many proposed reforms that the evidence demonstrates are clearly wrong.)

In practice, there is also a tendency to define our policy activities in dealing with equity in terms of sickness care rather than with broader determinants of health, such as having adequate food, shelter, and income. As one example, the Canadian Medical Association held a national dialogue on the social determinants of health but ended up suggesting that the most pressing need was to ensure "equitable access to effective and appropriate health care services."[6]

Access and Wait Times

Timely access to care has been one of the most persistent issues when discussing Canadian health care. How much waiting is acceptable? One positive impact of the focus on measuring and monitoring wait times is that considerable efforts have been made to try to standardize the findings and make sure we are comparing apples to apples. However, there is still considerable variability in what different reports examine; not surprisingly, the results may accordingly vary with who is reporting and on what.

One key access issue is whether people can find a primary care provider. As previously noted, there are still differences in the extent to which this happens, but it has been improving. One main factor affecting it is the type of health system. As noted in Chapter 3, Canada uses a public financing-private delivery (public contracting) model for physician services. This contrasts with the public financing-public delivery approach that Canada uses for public schools. If I move to a new home, my child is assigned to a school, a classroom, and a teacher. I do not get to choose which teacher my child will get; neither can the teacher decide whether she wants to admit my child to her class. Finding a physician is different. I do get to pick my family doctor (just as he or she also gets to choose whether to accept me). However, if I move, or if my doctor decides to retire, there is often no obvious way to connect me with a new one. A number of methods have been tried, but they may or may not work. As will be noted in Chapter 8, one approach that is being tried is to revise the models of primary care and de-emphasize solo practice. These new models may also be more attractive to physicians; running a solo practice can be extremely time-consuming, and younger physicians trying to balance their personal and professional lives understandably appear to be far less willing to work those many hours.

Within Canada, different provinces have tried various ways to connect people and primary care doctors. One option is to encourage rostering of patients to providers (as briefly described in Chapter 2). Clearly, any payment mechanism using rostering means, by definition, that once a physician agrees to roster me, I am that physician's patient. But finding a physician who is willing and able to take patients may be more complicated. A number of experiments have been tried. In Ontario, for example, Health Care Connect (started in 2009) allows people who have a valid OHIP card but do not currently have a family health care provider to register and get help in finding a local primary care provider who is willing to accept patients. The doctor, in turn, gets a one-time incentive payment for agreeing to take them; at the time of writing it still used the 2011 fee code of $350 for enrolling a new patient, plus an additional $500 if the patient was seen as being a "complex vulnerable patient." One consequence is, according to some sources, the number of patients without a primary care doctor in Ontario has dropped considerably.[7]

However, even having a doctor does not mean that I can easily get an appointment. One frequently used metric for system performance (heavily relied on by some international comparisons, including the Commonwealth Fund), is whether people can see their family doctor on the same or next day when they are sick. As we noted in Chapter 5, Canada ranks near the bottom on this metric. Results from the 2015 Commonwealth Fund survey of primary care physicians in 10 countries did find some improvement over time; 53% of Canadian doctors surveyed said that their patients could get same or next-day appointments, an increase from the 2009 figure (39%) but still much worse than most other countries being surveyed (average 72%).[8]

One possible work-around is to visit a walk-in clinic or an emergency department (ED) of the local hospital. This is usually considered suboptimal; such clinics or EDs don't have access to my patient records, which can hamper the efficiency of the visit, and these models are often a costlier way to deliver care. Another approach is to encourage primary care models to deliver after-hours care. As noted above, this may not be easy for solo practitioners, who cannot (and should not be expected to) work the number of hours that would be needed to provide such services. Increasingly, therefore, primary care models in many jurisdictions are encouraging group practice, which often includes non-physician health professionals on the team. These groups may allow the economies of scale associated with having staff available evenings and weekends in case their services might be needed while still allowing them to have a life outside of their medical practice. To the extent that a primary care model is already paying their providers for delivering after-hours care, the third-party payers may impose financial penalties on physicians whenever patients rostered to their practice seek care outside of it (e.g., in Ontario, they may claw back portions of the "access bonus" if their patients receive care from walk-in clinics or other family practitioners outside of their team). In theory, this should mean that doctors have a strong incentive to provide good after-hours care and to let their patients know how to access it. In practice, they may instead de-roster those patients who heavily rely on after-hours care (although they may still allow them to stay with their clinical practice, albeit on a FFS basis rather than as rostered patients); some have referred to this as firing the patient since, depending on the funding model, these patients would no longer be able to freely access the non-physician services that practice offered (e.g., consultations with dieticians).

Another access issue relates to wait times in hospital emergency rooms. The extent of such waiting depends on where you are going, when, and for what. Clearly, for a genuine emergency, the hospital is the best place to go. Even for less serious conditions, the hospital may still be the optimal place to go in many small communities, particularly in situations where the hospital emergency room would have to be staffed in case their services were needed but would not have many patients actually needing (and demanding) those services. In other communities, where hospitals are already very busy, relying on them would be suboptimal, often resulting in long waits to see a clinician, at a higher cost than seeking care elsewhere, and at a greater risk of information not flowing between the hospital and the other care providers in the community.

A related issue, which has also attracted considerable attention, is that of wait lists and wait times. How long must you wait to see a specialist or to receive a diagnostic procedure? How many people are waiting for care? What should be considered good performance? What are the implications of having to wait for care?

The potential solutions to wait times will depend on the reasons why these wait times exist. Accordingly, analysts often subdivide these reasons to distinguish between several phases of waiting. Most analyses start with the patient's decision to seek out care (although these may ignore the time that often passes between the beginning of symptoms and the patient's realization that care might be needed). Because primary care is usually the gatekeeper, we can then count how much time elapses between the primary care doctor referring the patient to a specialist and that consultation actually occurring. We can then measure how much time elapses between the patient seeing the specialist and the patient receiving the recommended treatment.

Deciding what is an appropriate wait time will vary depending on the circumstances. Some things clearly need immediate attention. Others might be scheduled at a time of mutual convenience. In the United Kingdom, for example, physicians were initially told that they would be evaluated on the basis of their ability to ensure that people could receive rapid access to primary care (specifically, seeing a professional within 24 hours and a primary care doctor within 48 hours). In turn, they found out that this policy inconvenienced people who needed a consultation but not immediately and who therefore wanted to book their appointments at a time convenient to them. I was told by one person that she was not allowed to do so but had to call in the morning for a same-day booking, since allowing her to book ahead of time would make the physicians look like they were imposing overly long wait times and adversely affect their evaluations. There were evidently enough similar complaints that they modified the model (in June 2010) and returned to the older policy of allowing people to book routine follow-up appointments at a mutually convenient time.[9] However, the potential for misleading indicators remains in any measurement system.

As we noted in Chapter 5, in many countries, including Canada, clinicians have attempted to set benchmarks that they can use to measure the quality of care. These benchmarks include how long it is appropriate to wait for different kinds of procedures. In 2004 as part of the Health Accord, Canada's provinces and territories set standards for maximum wait times for some specified procedures, based on the best evidence available at the time; these are sometimes called the pan-Canadian benchmarks. Canada's wait time strategy singled out a number of procedures: cancer radiation therapy, coronary artery by-pass surgery, diagnostic imaging (by MRI and CT), hip replacement and knee replacement, and cataract surgery. Why these particular procedures were selected is not always clear, but they provide a useful starting point. One problem with using them as a measure of performance is that these procedures vary widely in their susceptibility to inappropriate use. People are unlikely to receive cancer radiation therapy if they do not need it, but there is much more scope for doing diagnostic imaging that may not be clinically justified.

Although the original target for improving wait times in these selected areas was March 31, 2007, this strategy is an ongoing issue rather than a final fix. As previously noted, a number of bodies try to monitor how well Canada performs in meeting these wait time targets. They do so in a variety of ways and may also vary in how they collect the data and from whom. Some of their reports examine administrative data (which can capture what treatment is received by analysing the providers' billing data). Others may survey physicians and patients. Many of these bodies release yearly reports, which allow analysis of how much things have improved (or worsened) over time.

CIHI has been monitoring and publishing indicators on wait times for selected priority procedures; in 2016 it published its 11th annual report on this subject.[10] Unsurprisingly, CIHI found that the picture is mixed; however, the overall results were encouraging. For example, even though the number of surgeries being performed was increasing, for the most part wait times were not. Performance was not perfect, but CIHI estimated that about 80% of patients were receiving these selected priority surgical procedures within the benchmark times. However, not surprisingly, since Canada uses a private delivery model, the results varied by procedure, by province, and also within provinces. An individual patient's experience is thus likely to vary, depending in large part where (and from whom) the patient was seeking care.

Another monitoring body, the Wait Time Alliance, is associated with major doctors' associations across Canada. It also analyses data from provincial health ministries to assign grades to each province, although they note that different hospitals (and regions) tracked different things. The Wait Time Alliance has set its own benchmarks, which are shorter than those set by the provinces. (As one example, their benchmark for access to radiation therapy is 10 days, while the pan-Canadian standard is four weeks.) One result is that although the Alliance tried to assign grades for a wide variety of benchmarks covering many clinical areas, the data were often not available for the indicators it had chosen. Accordingly, the report showed insufficient data (which they denoted by assigning a grade of "?") for the majority of indicators in most provinces (Newfoundland and Labrador, for example, had no grades for 39 of the 43 benchmarks on the table).[11]

The OECD also analysed wait times. It compared Canada to six other countries (United Kingdom, Australia, New Zealand, Finland, Estonia, and Portugal); Canada ranked best in cataract surgery and second in hip and knee replacements.[12]

The Fraser Institute think tank surveys medical specialists and asks them how much time elapses between a patient being referred to them and that patient receiving treatment. Its 2015 report estimated that the wait time was just over 18 weeks; however, these numbers also varied considerably, both across provinces, and by specialty.[13]

As is clear by noting the diversity of reports, analysing what these wait times mean and how best to ensure that care is not jeopardized can be complicated. However, the various studies do make a number of suggestions about how best to reduce them. For example, the Wait Times Alliance pointed out that a number of factors were contributing to wait times, which in turn suggested a number of policy levers that could be used to help improve them.

Some of these related to inadequate resources (including people, equipment, operating room time, and beds) to deal with the existing demand. Dealing with these issues would require that increased resources be given to providers. In part, this would depend on how much demand there is for particular services, which may vary over time. For example, more patients are receiving radiation therapy; the number grew by 34% between 2010 and 2015. In turn, this requires careful attention to how many health care professionals we need and to issues around recruitment and retention to ensure that they are willing to work where they are needed. Reassuringly, the CIHI report found that 98% of patients Canada-wide were receiving their radiation therapy within the benchmark time.

Some of the problems with access appear to be related to suboptimal use of existing resources; these could be dealt with through better management. Some deal with poor coordination and bottlenecks; examples include people still occupying acute hospital beds because they are waiting for LTC, or people not getting care because they did not have a primary care provider. Fixing these problems requires better system integration of the various silos of care. Other wait time problems relate to inappropriate care that should not have been requested in the first place, which requires closer attention to implementing clinical guidelines for quality improvement.

Another question is the consequence of waiting and the impact on outcomes. Again, this will vary with the condition being analysed. Radiation therapy clearly needs to be given in a timely manner, but other services may be less essential. For example, although hip and knee replacement surgery can be very helpful to people with mobility problems, these may not be permanent fixes because some of the devices used in hip or knee replacement surgery wear out. In at least some cases, subsequent surgeries are less likely to be successful, and many surgeons try to avoid having to do too many revisions. Accordingly, there may be advantages to the patient in agreeing to wait until the surgery is needed to lessen how many subsequent procedures might be needed. Deciding when to do these kinds of elective procedures depends on the views and preferences of the patient, and on the procedure and its success rates. The CIHI report noted that the proportion meeting the target for some of these procedures was lower but still fairly good for hip fracture repair (87%), hip replacement (81%), knee replacement (77%), and cataract surgery (76%); no benchmarks had yet been established for bypass surgery, cancer surgery, CT scans, or MRI scans. A related problem was that hospitals faced with budgetary constraints might limit and prioritize their activities; elective surgery, however valuable, could lose out to what was considered more urgent uses of operating room time.

To the extent that the problems arise from inefficiencies within organizations, some hospitals have been working with system design experts to improve how they deliver care. For example, industrial engineers have long recognized that *queuing theory* can help reduce waiting times.[14] Queuing theory uses mathematical models to predict how long a person would have to wait and identify ways this might be changed. These models specify a number of variables, including the rate at which the "customers" requiring service arrive, the rate at which they are served (the "service time"), the number of servers in the system, and the manner in which the customers are selected from the queue for service (which is called the "queue discipline"). A variety of rules can be used for deciding how to do this selection. The most obvious, although not necessarily the most efficient, is first come–first served. Another alternative that is known to reduce the average wait time is to give priority to those who will need the lowest processing time; a common example is the "eight items or less" line seen in many supermarkets. However, using this approach will force the more complex customers to wait longer, which may work for grocery shoppers but could be problematic for health care. Another commonly used alternative (particularly in hospital emergency rooms) is to triage and see the most severe cases first, forcing the less complex cases to wait. A queuing theory analysis thus highlights potential ways to manage the queues; options include changing the queue discipline rules but also slowing the rate at which customers enter the system (or limiting how many can be waiting in the line), increasing the number of servers, and increasing how quickly a case can be served (the "service rate"). One of the simplest ways to do this is to have a single line, which means that instead of being stuck behind a complex case, you will be able to see the next available agent (or doctor). Banks and airports often adopt this approach, and it is increasingly being used in health care. One commonly used term is *pooled referral system*; for example, allowing patients to be seen by the next available surgeon rather than having to wait for a particular doctor. In the United Kingdom the NHS has found that this is a very useful way to reduce wait times. Saskatchewan has followed their lead; its "Putting the Patient First" surgical initiative allows patients to choose between asking to see a particular specialist and agreeing to see the next available specialist. This pooled model can be advantageous for both patients (whose wait time is reduced) and also for the specialists, since it provides them with a steady stream of referrals and cuts down on waste by ensuring that more available appointment slots are filled.[15]

Examining care processes and applying systems analysis tools can be extremely helpful in streamlining processes in many ways. One example was a hospital that claimed that it did not have enough recovery rooms; analysis of the patient flow revealed that the hospital was starting multiple surgical procedures in different operating rooms at the same time. By staggering the start times, the hospital was able to increase the number of surgeries that could be done, while making better use of the existing facilities; the hospital found it indeed did have enough recovery rooms.[16]

Quality of Care and Patient Safety

The other side of waiting times is *appropriateness*. If the patient does not need a procedure at all (or does not need it at this time), access can cause harm. This evokes some of the questions addressed in Chapter 6 about how much damage is being done to false positives. In 2012 a group of US physicians began a campaign they called Choosing Wisely, which has now spread to at least 15 other countries. Choosing Wisely Canada, which we discussed in Chapter 6, has been established in partnership with the Canadian Medical Association and the provincial and territorial medical associations. Its slogan is "More is not always better," and it has been identifying tests and procedures that their expert reviews conclude are not supported by the evidence. Recognizing that this is rarely a yes or no situation, its website, which provides informational material, by specialty, for patients and providers, often indicates the situations and categories of patients for which these selected interventions are or are not seen as necessary.[17]

Another key area of focus, which is attracting considerable attention, is improving quality of care. One example is what are sometimes called *adverse events*. Avoiding these is a clear example of win-win situations. If a hospital patient gets an infection, or is given the wrong medication (or wrong dose), the results are often worse outcomes at a higher cost. One key study, the 2004 Canadian Adverse Events Study, found that there was indeed a substantial burden of injury among hospital patients. Although it sparked a number of efforts to improve things, including establishing the Canadian Patient Safety Institute, progress has been slower than desired. One potential reason is the reluctance to report errors for fear of legal consequences. These improvement efforts involve a number of groups and approaches, including health professions regulatory bodies, accreditation procedures, more patient involvement, and better reporting and monitoring.[18] Some provinces have also set up provincial agencies with a mandate to monitor and improve quality. One example is Ontario, where the provincial government passed the *Excellent Care for All Act*, which requires health care organizations to establish quality committees, and report their findings to its provincial quality agency (Health Quality Ontario), but it has been criticized for its relative lack of public reporting.[19] Improving quality and avoiding errors where possible is a clear example of where all parties have similar interests. Efforts to identify and transfer best practices would seem an obvious area, and it is encouraging that more and more jurisdictions and organizations are recognizing that investing in these areas makes sense. This emphasis on monitoring and reporting is also linked to the emphasis on accountability.

Accountability

Considerable attention has been paid to the need to increase accountability in health care (and indeed, in many other policy areas). As we noted in a series of research projects examining accountability within subsectors in Ontario, and across Canada, there is increasing recognition that one size does not fit all and that it is important to unpack the concept to clarify what might work best under which circumstances.[20]

Accountability means having to be answerable; we must accordingly specify for what, by whom, to whom, and how (including the consequences for good or poor performance). The *for what* can include financial, performance, and political or democratic dimensions.[21] Within health care, this may translate into fiscal accountability to payers for how their money is spent; clinical accountability to regulators, providers, and patients for the quality of care; and accountability to the public. The mechanisms used may include a variety of policy instruments, as noted in Chapter 1.

We found that particular emphasis was being placed on three of these policy instruments. Financial incentives use the expenditure instrument, sometimes in the form of *pay for performance*. Regulations are commonly employed to require various forms of activity by health care providers; the *to whom* element includes an array of actors, including payers, professional regulators, and accreditation bodies. There is also considerable use of the exhortation instrument, both in the form of information directed towards patients and payers (including posting report cards) and in the form of relying on professionalism and the desire of providers to do the right thing for their patients. There was also considerable variation in the rewards and punishments associated with meeting (or not meeting) performance targets. For example, if people or organizations do not meet targets because of inadequate resources, should they be given more money or staff? If so, how do we avoid setting up incentives for failure?

Public reporting is often accompanied by "shame and blame" to those identified as being relatively poor performers. This may provide incentives to improve but may lead to reluctance to monitor performance at all. This tension has been an ongoing issue in the patient safety movement, where providers worried about the possibility of being sued and had an incentive to cover up errors. The quality improvement movement has made great strides in encouraging what is usually called a *culture of safety*; this includes reporting, not only of actual errors, but also of near misses that did not lead to a poor outcome but might have.[22] Examination of such events has in turn helped to identify the factors that caused these problems to occur, and ideally to implement changes that will help minimize such problems in the future. These patient safety initiatives are usually coupled with a policy of mandatory reporting to patients; rather than spark lawsuits (as feared), the evidence suggests that such reporting has often been shown to increase patients' trust in their providers and to improve care.

In the research projects noted above, we found that the extent to which these different accountability approaches succeeded depended heavily on a number of factors, including the goals of the exercise, the governance or ownership structures in place (which affected both who would be accountable to whom and the sorts of policy levers available), and on the characteristics of the activities being conducted. In particular, we looked at the impact of the *production characteristics'* we discussed in Chapter 3.

The goals of accountability exercises varied but often included combinations of ensuring access, quality (including safety), satisfaction, and cost control or cost-effectiveness. Difficulties often ensued when these goals conflicted. The governance or ownership structures in place also raised a number of issues. Private for-profit organizations, for example, have an obligation to maximize the return to their shareholders, which may affect which sorts of services they offer and to whom. Although physicians may be faced with similar incentives, as "not only for profit" organizations they usually focus on trying to ensure that they help their patients.

We found that the production characteristics of the services being provided did play a critical role. In particular, there was a tendency to focus on things that were easy to measure, even when these were not the most important outcomes. Factors less easy to measure were often ignored. Another key finding was that organizations were reluctant to be held responsible for things they could not control. For example, tobacco use may be an important determinant of health, but if providers cannot control whether their patients smoke, they may be reluctant to be accountable for, and potentially penalized for, how often their patients decide to light up a cigarette. This also proved important internationally in attempts to introduce performance measurement.[23] As one example, public health units serving poorer neighbourhoods were cautious about what metrics should be included in their accountability arrangements and tended to avoid those which dealt with population health, even though such factors were critical influences on the health outcomes in that jurisdiction.[24]

These concerns about being accountable for things not under our control also influenced the tendency to avoid looking at what happens when care crosses silos. Who is responsible for ensuring smooth transitions between hospitals and home or community? How do we manage the hand-offs to primary care? These issues of service integration (and the lack thereof) recur as significant barriers to performance, albeit ones that tend to be ignored in many accountability systems.

The former Health Council of Canada published a report evaluating the results of the health care reform agenda set out in the 2004 Accord. It concluded that the impact had been limited. Although some improvements had indeed occurred in certain areas (including wait times, primary care reform, drug coverage, and use of electronic health records), there were still health inequities. The report relied heavily on the Commonwealth Fund data and emphasized the importance of pursuing the triple aim objectives of better health, better care, and better value. They concluded that the emphasis had primarily been on care, with insufficient attention to whether these investments improved overall health and provided value for money. The Health Council called for placing more emphasis on pan-Canadian collaboration to try to ensure that each jurisdiction would have comparable results. It viewed leadership, at all levels, as the key lever and noted the difficulty in maintaining policy directions when governments changed.[25] Ironically, the Council itself became an example of this point; it had been set up as an arm's-length body in 2003 by the Liberal government as part of the Health Accords with the provinces, with the mandate to facilitate public reporting on health reform and disseminating information about best practices. However, after the federal government changed, its funding was not renewed by the Harper government in 2014 on the grounds that it had completed its mandate.[26]

In the final chapter, I return to the reform suggestions noted in the Introduction of this book.

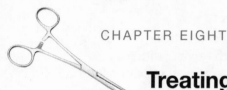

CHAPTER EIGHT

Treating Health Care: How Can We Make It Better? What Might Make It Worse?

Having attempted to describe and diagnose Canadian health care, I will focus in this chapter on a number of potential treatments for what ails it. Fortunately, the diagnosis suggests that health care is not terminally ill, but there is clearly room for improvement. However, some treatment suggestions are likely to make things worse.

The data shown in Chapter 4 (Figure 4.1) outlining the distribution of health expenditures suggest two obvious policy directions to examine. First, can we keep those who are not currently using many resources (the "low spenders") healthy? This would point to the need to focus on the determinants of health and ensure that most of the population would be able to enjoy healthy lives for as long as possible. Second, can we examine the care being given to the small proportion of people who account for so much of the health care bill, and see whether we have ways to make this care more cost-effective? Building on some of the concepts and background information described in earlier chapters, I here try to see what they might imply for the reform suggestions noted in the Introduction. Underlying them all is the need to recognize that health care involves dealing with people and the importance of ensuring that they should all (and always) be respected as individuals. The suggestions I will discuss are as follows:

- Make people healthier and help them stay healthy.
- Improve how services are coordinated (service integration) and improve the quality of care.

- Change how we organize our system, including revisiting how we pay for care (including who pays for what) and how we deliver it (including doing something about wait lists and access).
- Become more efficient, to get better value for money.

Make People Healthier

One obvious win-win possibility is to keep people healthier. This is a desirable outcome; very few people enjoy being in pain, having their movements restricted, having to have surgery, or having to take medications. It may also save money if we can reduce the amount of care that people need.

As noted in Chapter 1, a number of important factors help determine how healthy we are. These include income and social status, education and literacy, employment and working conditions, the physical environment (including air and water quality), but also personal relationships (including our social support networks and the social environment we live in), and our personal health practices and social skills. A focus on the determinants of health will in turn suggest a number of potential action steps. We could focus on various combinations of growing the economy and improving income levels, improving education, modifying the built environment (including encouraging more walkable communities), encouraging healthy eating (including requiring clearer food labelling), providing high-quality child care, addressing air pollution, improving housing and making it more affordable, encouraging people to plant community gardens, increasing wage levels, reducing crime rates, and so on.[1] One potential focus is to start with children and ensure they are well fed, well housed, and well educated, and participate in healthy behaviours (including eating well, exercising, and being engaged in their community). As noted in the discussion of the determinants of health, addressing such issues are key but how to do so is complex and multifaceted and extends far beyond the health care system. Some of the proposed interventions are likely to be contentious, particularly to the extent that they involve reconciling different ideas about the roles of government and the community (e.g., how much should we expect people to pay to help others, how much should we restrict people's freedom of action).

If we restrict our attention to secondary or tertiary prevention, we may want to focus on better care management, which may include helping educate those with chronic conditions about how to minimize the complications arising from their conditions. Much of this links with the next reform suggestion, to improve how we integrate services and ease transitions of care across care providers (where providers may also include patients and their families).

Improve How Services Are Coordinated (Service Integration) and the Quality of Care

One obvious area for improvement, as noted in Chapter 6, is to improve the quality of care and patient safety. This may not always be easy but is not very contentious. Few would argue in favour of having patients get avoidable infections, giving them the wrong medications, or operating on the wrong patients. Patient safety is – and remains – an ongoing focus of most providers. Although most providers do a fairly good job, most would also agree that the ideal – no mistakes at all – is difficult to achieve, which does not mean that they do not keep trying to do better.

A more difficult reform is improving service integration. As noted in Chapter 7, a number of the strategies associated with improving access (including reducing wait times) relate to this. One major problem is that health care is often delivered in silos.[2] In effect, care is usually organized around the providers rather than around the patients. Care may be very high quality within each of those silos, but the system (or non-system) can present major problems when people transition among providers. A clear example is what happens when people are discharged from hospital. Who is responsible for ensuring that the necessary care is delivered once that patient leaves the building? Who is responsible for ensuring that information about diagnoses, tests, and medications flows to where it is needed? These needs for coordination become particularly important for people with *multiple morbidities*, a term used to describe people with more than one chronic health problem. (The term *co-morbidity* is sometimes used to describe the same situation.) Dealing with someone as "a diabetic," for example, may ignore the fact that the person also has cardiac problems or high blood pressure.[3] Without good care coordination, these patients may have a much worse quality of life, as well as being more expensive to treat (e.g., if they have to go to hospital emergency rooms rather than be managed in the community). Ideally, their care will be well managed, keeping their blood pressure and blood sugar well enough controlled that they do not have urgent health problems, but in too many cases people are overlooked.

A number of efforts are underway to try to improve these care coordination processes; they address a wide array of goals and thus may select from a wide array of potential tools. As discussed earlier, some of these efforts emphasize the importance of what is often termed *patient-centred care* and stress such goals as ensuring that information is available to those who need it (including patients and their families), that the information is clear and culturally relevant, and that people can be involved in choosing what they want and need. Patient-centred care may also mean shifting activities from providers to patients (often spoken of as the need to empower patients and have them care for themselves), which may reduce costs to providers and payers, but may or may not benefit patients and their caregivers, depending on how willing and able they are to take on those responsibilities.

Scholars have noted that the integration of care can have multiple meanings. What is sometimes called *functional integration* relates to organizations and means that they coordinate key activities (including financial management so providers don't have to fill out multiple sets of forms, or information management so that the electronic health records can talk to one another). This will rarely affect patients directly but will help ensure that the organizations from which they seek care operate more smoothly. Another definition relates to *physician integration*, which deals with how physicians are linked into a system of care. In terms of improving patient care, the emphasis is heavily on what is often called *clinical integration*, which means that there is 'continuity of care' and good communication among providers. This can represent a win-win by doing things like eliminating duplicate testing and procedures, and ensuring that things don't fall through the cracks when people move from one provider to another. This approach will usually entail elements of inter-professional collaboration and reduced barriers to access. One common theme of all these efforts is the need to improve care transitions as people move across care silos and ensure continuity of care.

A wide variety of mechanisms to accomplish this care integration have been suggested. Two that have received particular attention involve changes to how care is organized and to the information technology that is being used. These approaches are not mutually exclusive; indeed, they can reinforce each other.

In terms of how care is organized, one major approach is to have an identified body that is responsible for patients and ensures that providers across the spectrum of care are linked. Primary care providers are frequently suggested as the most appropriate group to take on this role. In turn, this usually requires knowing who is responsible for each patient. A frequent approach is to ensure that all patients are linked or rostered with an identified primary care provider (as discussed earlier). It will often include introducing care models that employ a wide variety of health care providers (including nurses, social workers, and dietitians), and, depending on the population being served, having primary care linked with groups that can address some of the social determinants of health. For example, some community health centres that manage care for vulnerable populations have links with social housing, legal aid, and similar services. We may also target groups with particular health issues and set up specialized organizations that can address their needs across the continuum of care; an example is setting up special programs to care for people with developmental delays.

Another major approach is to take advantage of the great advances in information technology to facilitate communication. Computerized records go by a number of names, including electronic medical records and electronic health records (EHR); I will use the term EHR. These were initially seen as a quick fix but have proven to be far more complex than initially envisioned. Ideally, a good EHR would ensure that patient information was accurately captured in a standardized format and shared with all those needing that information (including both the patient and those treating that patient). This would prevent patients having to repeat information and tests, and would ensure that updates to patient records would be sent in a timely manner. Some of these goals have indeed been achieved. Others have not or have been partially successful.

One complexity relates to who should be using the EHRs (and who should have access to them). Ideally, we would ensure that primary care, hospitals, pharmacies, and laboratory tests, at minimum, used compatible systems. In that case, whenever a patient went into a hospital (or a hospital emergency room), the information would be sent to their primary care provider, as well as to the relevant specialists. Rather than the patient having to take the prescription to the pharmacist, the EHR would send it to the pharmacist directly, would check it against other prescriptions that patient is receiving and against other co-morbidities, and alert physicians and pharmacists to potential medication errors. The EHR would alert providers (and patients) to critical laboratory results. It would even send key information to public health as required (e.g., if the laboratory results indicated that the patient had a reportable communicable disease). By replacing paper charts, EHRs could allow physicians to obtain, interpret, and act on information without having to be physically present in that facility and free up space in the office that would otherwise be devoted to filing cabinets. EHRs might also highlight the need to ensure that data are accurately captured and improve the quality of records. (One of the first laws of computers was GIGO, which stands for "garbage in, garbage out"; good EHRs would presumably minimize the amount of bad information being captured.)

In practice, however, a number of issues have arisen. First, the systems can be expensive. Also, in the absence of central mandates, different providers may be using different systems, which may or may not communicate well with one another. Important information may be difficult (and time-consuming) to enter. People may take the lazy way out and cut and paste previous material, even if it is no longer accurate. Available codes in the EHR may not accurately capture the nuances of a particular patient. Privacy concerns may mean that information sharing should be controlled; having this information in electronic records may even present some risk of identity theft. New systems may require constant updating. Without backups, a computer crash can lead to data loss.

Nonetheless, improving EHR (including improving the quality of the data these records attempt to capture), and therefore ensuring that key information is available in a timely manner to those who need it, is an obvious area for improvement.[4]

Change How We Organize Our System

The next set of reform suggestions relates to changing how we organize our system, including revisiting how we pay for care (including who pays for what) and how we deliver it (including doing something about wait lists and access). These proposed reforms are an interesting mix of things that might make things better and things that the evidence strongly suggests would make things worse. Here, clearly defining our terms is essential. For example, although some argue that Canada should end the public monopoly on delivering care, Chapter 4 clarified that this description of the status quo is not accurate. Canada does not use public delivery; it uses a public contracting model where delivery is private (or, in the case of the services delivered by regional health authorities in some provinces, is quasi-public). There is accordingly no need to end a public monopoly on delivering care in Canada, since Canada does not have one to eliminate. Financing, in contrast, is indeed public for those interventions meeting the definition of insured services for insured persons but not for the increasing array of medically necessary care that is delivered outside of hospitals by non-physician providers.

Changing Financing: How Should We Pay for Care?

As noted in Chapter 2, we have a large number of silos of health care. Deciding who should pay for what is an obvious, and ongoing, area for debate. As noted in Chapter 4, Canada requires full public payment for all insured health services to all insured persons, but this applies only if this care is provided in a hospital or by a physician. Provincial and territorial insurance plans can go beyond this but are not required to do so. There have been suggestions to change this, some of which argue for decreasing what the public pays for and others for expansion of the list of insured services.

Allowing Private Payment

One frequent fear is that a system relying heavily on publicly funded care will not be sustainable. Canada's current financing model leaves no scope for allowing insured persons to pay privately for insured services. One suggestion – which I would argue is a clear example of a bad idea – is to relax this requirement. Such proposals take several major forms, which are not mutually exclusive.

One approach would impose user fees (which could be in the form of co-payments or deductibles), often working on the assumption that having people pay would reduce moral hazard and thereby reduce waste by ensuring that people do not use services they would not deem worth paying for. Canada does permit user fees for insured persons but only for care not seen to be medically necessary, as well as for those services not encompassed by the CHA definition of insured services. Those proposing that user fees also be permitted for hospital and physician care often note that most other countries do incorporate co-pays as part of their coverage (but do not inform us that they have a wider definition of insured services than Canada does; as Table 5.1 showed, this nets out to a higher – not lower – proportion of health costs being paid for from public sources in most of these other jurisdictions than in Canada). The evidence is clear that user fees can indeed discourage people from seeking care, but this effect is not very sensitive to whether that care is necessary. If necessary care is not used, then as noted earlier we may end up with worse health outcomes and higher total costs; consider the example of people who have a stroke because they could not afford medication to reduce their blood pressure. User fees also tend to lead to higher total prices, because individual patients do not have the same bargaining power as larger purchasers to negotiate fees. User fees may even encourage unnecessary and inappropriate treatments if the facility has excess capacity and wants to use it. Indeed, Canadian health economist Robert Evans has called user fees for necessary care an example of "zombies" – ideas that should have been killed off but keep coming back to life to do damage.[5]

A related model would replace insurance coverage with *medical savings accounts* (MSAs). Under these models, individuals (or families) would be given a lump sum of money, which they could use to directly purchase health care services, rather than having the costs covered by third-party payers. Models vary. One question is how much would be given and by whom (some of these models would eliminate government-paid insurance in favour of government providing or subsidizing the lump sum payments to individual MSAs; others would have the money paid by employers and by tax-subsidized payments by individuals). Other sources of variation include whether funds not spent could be accumulated (i.e., whether "use it or lose it" applies) and whether these MSAs would be supplemented with catastrophic insurance for severe illness. Basically, the MSA model eliminates risk pooling for those services to be covered by the MSAs. In theory, this would reduce moral hazard and make people more conscious of their spending.

In practice, this is not what happens. As Figure 4.1 in Chapter 4 showed, health care costs tend to be heavily skewed. Those who have examined the distribution of health expenditures have found that the majority of the population is almost always relatively healthy. If the funds are intended to purchase care that one would not want unless it was needed, most of the money would be wasted (although it might make a reassuring increase in those people's bank accounts). In contrast, there would usually be insufficient funds to cover the costs of those with high needs, leaving them with catastrophic expenditures or the inability to purchase needed care. In a study with Forget and Roos, our analysis of MSAs internationally concluded that these models usually represent high costs for minimal benefit.[6]

Another possibility is to allow two-tier coverage, in which patients would still be eligible to receive free care from their publicly funded coverage but could pay extra (either out of pocket or through buying supplementary private insurance) to receive a higher level of care. For that extra money, they might get prompter treatment (sometimes called *jumping the queue*), treatment from a different doctor who does not participate in the publicly funded system, or a nicer room. Some argue that this would relieve the pressure on the publicly funded system, since those willing to pay more to use the private tier would therefore exit the public tier, which would also mean shorter wait times for those remaining in the public tier. It sounds like a win-win. It isn't. The international evidence is conclusive that most efforts to introduce two-tier health care can be seen as a lose-lose; total costs are higher, and wait times (and often quality of care) in the publicly funded sector are worse. There are several explanations. First, people have no reason to enter the private tier unless what they could get in the publicly funded sector is inadequate (or perceived to be inadequate). In addition, clinicians have strong incentives to shift as much of their practice as they can to private patients. Costs to the public plan may indeed go down, but this is a result of cost shifting rather than cost savings. To the extent that employers are expected to pay some of these costs through their benefits plans, it also erodes the economic competitiveness of that jurisdiction.[7]

Indeed, in 2002, the Canadian Senate report (Kirby Committee) explicitly addressed the question of whether the current system was fiscally sustainable. In section 1.1.3, it wrote: "The Committee is keenly aware that shifting more of the cost to individual patients and their families via private payments, the facile 'solution' recommended by many, is really nothing more than an expensive way of relieving or, at the least, diminishing governments' problem. Regardless of how it is expressed (as a share of GDP, share of government spending, etc.), there is only one source of funding for health care – the Canadian public – and it has been shown conclusively that the most cost-effective way of funding health care is by using a single (in our case, publicly administered or governmental) insurer/payer model."[8] An identical recommendation was made by the Romanow Commission; its final report included the following:

> Early in my mandate, I challenged those advocating radical solutions for reforming health care – user fees, medical savings accounts, de-listing services, greater privatization, a parallel private system – to come forward with evidence that these approaches would improve and strengthen our health care system. The evidence has not been forthcoming. I have also carefully explored the experiences of other jurisdictions with co-payment models and with public-private partnerships, and have found these lacking. There is no evidence these solutions will deliver better or cheaper care, or improve access (except, perhaps, for those who can afford to pay for care out of their own pockets). More to the point, the principles on which these solutions rest cannot be reconciled with the values at the heart of medicare or with the tenets of the Canada Health Act that Canadians overwhelmingly support. It would be irresponsible of me to jeopardize what has been, and can remain, a world-class health care system and a proud national symbol by accepting anecdote as fact or on the dubious basis of making a "leap of faith."[9]

A related issue is whether we should encourage a greater role for *competition and choice*, which often is interpreted as meaning a larger role for for-profit (FP) delivery instead of public, NFP, or not-only-for-profit delivery. This is highly controversial. Some argue that market forces can encourage competition, which will improve efficiency. Sometimes that may indeed be the case, particularly where there are possibilities of economies of scale (especially for services that could span jurisdictional boundaries) or better management. However, others note that there is no clear reason why FP providers would be better positioned to make those savings and even less reason why policy should encourage those savings to be translated into profits for shareholders rather than used for other purposes. Because FP organizations will often deliver a different mix of services than their public or NFP competitors, such comparisons are difficult. For example, FP organizations rarely serve rural or remote communities, or populations without the income to pay for enhanced services.

In particular, the international evidence strongly suggests that FP organizations will attempt to focus on potentially profitable services and client groups, leaving less profitable groups that still need care to be served by public or NFP providers. We must also see how the savings are made and whether these measures are considered desirable. (Obvious possibilities for decreasing their costs beyond risk selection or cream skimming include changing wage levels and skill mixes of those providing the services and sacrificing difficult-to-measure intangibles, such as spending more time talking to patients.) As noted in Chapter 3, the production characteristics of the goods and services are important; the literature strongly suggests that NFP delivery tends to be superior when measurability is poor, as well as when contestability is low. NFP providers appear to be less sensitive to bottom-line incentives and hence more likely to deliver higher quality of care under these circumstances.

Another issue is the role for competition. For competition to exist, there must usually be excess capacity (or low barriers for new providers to enter the market); otherwise, the competing providers would not be able to take on the additional cases. This does not mean that we must remain with the status quo. If the status quo does not sufficiently ensure that patient needs and demands are responded to, it may be necessary to explore other mechanisms to make sure this happens.

One interesting development has been observed in situations that can be seen as quasi-monopolies – that is, where there are high barriers to entry and not enough work to keep multiple providers in business. Under those circumstances, competition has often proven problematic. One possibility that has often been seen was that FP companies would initially give low bids to drive out their competitors but then increase their prices once they had a monopoly. An example was garbage collection, where private companies initially looked like cost-effective alternatives to public provision but in the end turned out to be far more expensive. Similar examples abound; for example, in the United States, costs of purchasing hospital services from for-profit hospitals were 8% to 24% higher, even with similar cost structures, because the FP hospitals were better at maximizing their reimbursements. In nursing homes, the FP facilities did reduce their costs but on average did so by providing lower quality care.[10]

As noted in Chapter 4, at present, the CHA requires the federal government to withhold transfer payments for provinces that force people to pay for services which fall within the definition of insured services. That makes this policy change less attractive (which the evidence suggests is a good thing). However, as some policy analysts have noted, to enforce the CHA conditions, the federal government must be both willing and able to do so. In turn, that means that the CHA cash contribution must remain sufficiently large, since tax points cannot be taken back even if the province does not comply with these rules. In that connection, another proposal, not currently on the table but floated in the past by some Conservative government advisers, was to convert all of the federal transfer to tax points. This would have allowed the federal government to announce a tax cut (although provincial governments would have needed to announce tax increases if they had wanted to use this tax room). This policy, should it ever be implemented, would make the CHA unenforceable, and, since tax points cannot be taken back, could not be reversed by subsequent governments. It would be a simple way to kill any national standards for health care in Canada, should anyone want to do so.

In summary, although Scrooge (before his visits from the three ghosts) might approve of increasing private payment for necessary care, few others would. These proposed reforms are likely to increase total costs (although not necessarily the share paid for publicly), make health status worse, and have particularly adverse effects on the most vulnerable members of the population. In my opinion, this is a clear example of a reform that should be avoided.

Changing Coverage: Who Should Pay for What?

In contrast, another reform suggestion argues for expanding what is publicly insured through expanding what is defined as an insured service. A key health policy issue is and remains how best to ensure that people have access to the treatments and products they need at a price they can afford. In turn, this means that some mechanism will have to be established to determine both what is needed (which would include for whom and under what circumstances) and what will or will not be paid for. One trend that has galvanized this is the recognition that, as care moves outside hospitals, the costs can accordingly be shifted from public to private payment. Although many of the studies that have looked at health care in Canada have suggested that medically necessary care should be covered regardless of where (or by whom) it is delivered, action has been slow.

Several services falling outside the insured services definition have received particular attention. One reform, frequently referred to as *pharmacare*, would improve coverage for necessary pharmaceuticals delivered outside hospitals.[11] Policy analysts note that Canada is the only country with universal health care coverage that does not include medically necessary outpatient pharmaceuticals. This policy problem can in turn be decomposed into several distinct but related issues.

One issue is pricing: some pharmaceuticals are extremely expensive, and they are becoming more so. This evokes the issues of what is worth buying and at what cost noted in Chapter 6. Because drugs involve intellectual property, they can be patented, which means that no one can compete with that product until the patent expires (in Canada, this is 20 years). When it does, competitors can produce generic versions of the product and sell them for less, should they judge that the market is sufficient to allow them to make a profit at that price. However, should the market not be large enough, or the product be seen as sufficiently necessary, producers can also increase the price they charge to far beyond what it costs them to make it. One example that attracted considerable publicity in 2016 was the high increases in the charges for EpiPens in the United States. The product, which is used to combat life-threatening allergic reactions and has a shelf life of only one year, is no longer under patent, but pharmaceutical company Mylan (which was the only company producing that product in the United States) hiked the price for a pack of two injectors from $83 to $600. In Canada, the product was distributed by a different company, Pfizer, and being sold for about $100, whereas in England it sold for about $69. Mylan's reaction to the resulting outrage was that it was running a business, and hence should be able to maximize their profit, although they did subsequently agree to produce a generic version at only triple the former price.[12]

As discussed in Chapters 4 and 6, who is in charge of deciding drug policy is complex. In Canada, approving drugs as being sufficiently safe and effective to be allowed on the market is deemed to be a federal responsibility. However, paying for them is left to provincial and territorial insurance plans and to private payers. In addition in 1987, Canada's federal government established the Patented Medicine Prices Review Board (PMPRB), a national agency that has a limited ability to control the prices that are charged for drugs. This independent body, albeit nominally under the jurisdiction of the federal minister of health, can review the prices that pharmaceutical companies are allowed to charge for their patented products. The PMPRB also has the power to hold public hearings and order the prices to be reduced should it find the prices to be excessive, although this power is limited to the price charged by the pharmaceutical company; wholesalers or pharmacies are not bound by these rules. Neither does it have any control over non-patented drugs, including generic products. The PMPRB also reports on pharmaceutical trends to assist policymakers. The formula used by the PMPRB to set the price, however, requires that it be set as the "median" of the prices being charged to Canada's "comparator countries" of France, Germany, Italy, Sweden, Switzerland, the United Kingdom, and the United States. In general, this means that Canada pays higher prices than many other OECD countries, since it cannot set a price at the low end of the scale. Because so many countries decided to regulate their drug prices based on what others were paying, the pharmaceutical companies developed an ingenious strategy. They publish artificially high prices that are used by the regulatory bodies, and then offer secret deals to those with better negotiating power. Because these reduced prices are secret, they do not affect what price others must pay.[13] Some international trade agreements also provide greater market power to the manufacturers, further reducing the ability for payers to save money on purchasing these products.

A related issue arises from the fact that those purchasing the products have less market power than would be the case if they were representing larger populations; even for the publicly paid for drugs (including those dispensed in hospitals and those that provincial governments have decided to cover), the individual provinces have relatively small populations and hence have far less bargaining power than bigger countries. In addition, the trend towards personalized medicine, which means smaller potential markets for each product, allows companies to charge even higher prices for each of them. One interesting development was the Pan-Canadian Pharmaceutical Alliance, a voluntary collaboration set up in 2010 by the provincial and territorial governments, which allows them to work together for greater bargaining power and to negotiate lower prices. In 2015 the new federal Liberal government agreed to join this alliance. The impact, to date, has been modest; a government press release indicated that the Alliance had "completed more than 89 negotiations on brand name drugs and achieved price reductions on 14 generic drugs," for a savings estimated at "more than $490 million annually."[14] To place that amount into perspective, CIHI estimated total spending on outpatient prescription drugs in 2015 was about $29.2 billion, of which about $12.6 billion was being paid through public plans. (Of the remaining $16.6 billion, about 60% was paid by private insurance, and the remaining 40% by individuals out of pocket.) Indeed, the private insurers have recently suggested that they should also be part of the bargaining arrangements so that they too could share in any price reductions.

Another issue affecting pharmacare is appropriateness: as discussed in Chapter 6, providers are working to improve prescribing behaviour and ensure that prescribed treatments are likely to do more good than harm. The evidence strongly suggests that unnecessary prescriptions can have negative (and expensive) health impacts. Certainly, the frequent "ask your doctor" commercials seen on television do not help, even though the announcer is usually kind enough to rapidly tell us all the complications these products may cause. One key resource is health technology assessment, which may give some sense of value for money. Another potentially important resource is the Choosing Wisely Canada initiative described in Chapter 6, which is trying to work with doctors and patients to clarify some of the areas of overuse. Similarly, there have been efforts to ensure that EHRs help alert physicians and pharmacists to potential areas of drug interactions and other areas where prescribing might be improved.

In Canada the federal government has responsibility for regulating drugs but not in deciding which ones will be paid for other than for the sub-populations who have at least some federal coverage (including First Nations, the military, veterans, prisoners, and federal employees). This puts pressure on provincial budgets, as people push for having coverage for all approved drugs. One consequence, as already noted, is that Canada pays more for drugs than many other countries do, leaves people with high out-of-pocket costs, and has too many people not filling prescriptions because they cannot afford them, often leading to the lose-lose situation of worse health outcomes at higher cost (e.g., people having strokes because they cannot afford medications to control blood pressure). Negotiations for a new Health Accord have suggested that the federal government might add money for pharmacare to its transfers, although this was not part of the federal offer made in 2016. Should this become part of a subsequent agreement, there is a strong possibility of a win-win, particularly given research suggesting that a universal public drug plan could reduce the total costs of purchasing prescription drugs by billions of dollars per year, as long as careful attention is paid to pricing and appropriateness.[15]

A similar set of issues arises when looking at paying for LTC, which as previously noted includes both institutional care and care in the home and community. How should we handle an aging population who may not have informal caregivers willing and able to help them? Should they be hospitalized because, although not acutely ill, it is unclear whether it would be safe for them to live alone in their home? Should we assume they will move to residential facilities (nursing homes or retirement homes)? Should we help them stay at home, and if so, what sort of help will they (and their caregivers) receive? Who should pay for it?

As noted in Chapter 2, LTC can be divided into three categories: acute care substitution, long-term care substitution, and prevention/maintenance. Ontario is an example of a province trying to improve home and community care; its policies had initially tried to emphasize all three categories of LTC. However, efforts to control costs, particularly efforts to facilitate sending people home as soon as they could be safely discharged from hospital, led Ontario's publicly funded home care programs to become focused almost entirely on acute care substitution. Patients who are occupying a hospital bed but no longer require the intensity of resources provided there are often referred to as ALC (alternate level of care). Ontario's model thus tried to ensure that such ALC patients being discharged from hospitals would receive publicly financed home care services through their local CCACs for a limited period to facilitate an earlier discharge. The other categories of clients could still access home care services but would have to pay for them themselves. This in turn points to the need to decide what we think should be publicly subsidized. A recent review of potential reform directions suggested that the inability to perform IADL (e.g., preparing meals, using transportation, using the telephone) was a main reason seniors were being sent to residential LTC.[16] Better access to community-based services could certainly delay such admissions. However, since LTC includes food and shelter (which tend not to be considered health care), in most cases people do have to pay for such services out of pocket. For example, in Ontario, regulated LTC beds cost about $160 per day, of which the user is expected to pay about $57 per day to cover the costs of room and board (the rest, which is publicly subsidized, includes services such as nursing care).

Similarly, we could discuss the extent to which publicly funded coverage should be expanded to cover other services, including dental care, vision care, rehabilitation, and mental health services. Notably, the 2016 federal/provincial discussions about renewing the health transfers have included offers of increased federal funding as long as it would be targeted at home care and to mental health. It is likely that these discussions will persist, and policies will vary depending on who holds power and which stories about individuals have gained public attention. Deciding what should be publicly covered and for whom does not have a single right answer; it depends on our views about solidarity and the relative responsibilities of people, their families and friends, and the broader society.

Changing How We Pay Providers

Another reform direction involves changing how we pay providers. This involves the concepts around allocation discussed in Chapter 3 and the incentives inherent in different payment models. As noted earlier, which model is best depends on a variety of factors, including whether we want to encourage providers to do more (if we think the quality problem is underuse) or to do less (if there are problems with overuse), as well as the cost structures associated with the care they are delivering. In most countries, there are continuing disputes between payers and providers regarding the best way to handle payment models. Since there is no single answer, these battles are likely to continue.

At the time of writing, some payers have been trying to make their costs more predictable; in turn, this has led many of them to try to replace FFS with bundled payments for a particular episode of care (or for caring for a patient). In addition, some payers have tried to reduce their costs through cutting hospital budgets, freezing fee schedules, and similar measures; these may result in longer wait times and other problems related to access to care. In general, these efforts tend to worsen relationships between payers and providers without being remarkably effective. Physicians may threaten to leave the jurisdiction, wait times may grow, and despite these measures costs may not even be well contained. Where possible, partnerships among payers, providers, and patients to encourage appropriateness, discourage overtreatment, and otherwise seek out win-win situations seem more likely to be helpful in the long term, but making it happen is not always easy.

In that connection, there are a number of policy issues relating to how we organize care. Should we fund care based on the service? The organization? The region? Who happens to be enrolled in a particular health network? Deciding which services should be regionalized and how funds flow can be complex, particularly if people do not receive their care in the region where they live. Sometimes, moving across regional boundaries is clinically advisable, particularly for those services where quality has been found to be associated with performing at least a minimal volume of those procedures. Sometimes it is just a matter of convenience, particularly if the boundaries do not correspond to where people would seek care. Canada uses a wide variety of models; these depend on the service, the province, and even the location within that province. Each seem to have advantages and disadvantages.

A number of reforms to payment models are possible, but careful attention to details is essential to ensure that there is net benefit. This will depend on many factors and is likely to be highly contentious, particularly since any of these models are likely to have winners and losers. To the extent possible, it would seem desirable to encourage payers, providers, and citizens to work together to ensure that the balance best fits the local situation and needs.

Changing Delivery

As noted earlier, we can also seek to revise models of care delivery. This has been particularly evident in primary care, which is moving away from solo practice towards more integrated and comprehensive models. The earlier suggestions about improving care integration are likely to be helpful. Similarly, encouraging care to be delivered in the most appropriate location is likely to improve quality and cut costs. For example, efforts to improve discharge planning, encourage care in the community (rather than in hospitals), and support family caregivers for people to remain at home are likely to be helpful. New electronic devices can allow people to monitor key indicators from home, transmitting the information to the relevant specialist and allowing problems to be detected before they cause major complications while decreasing the need to physically travel for care. There are a number of current examples; these include devices that allow people with diabetes to monitor their blood glucose, people with hypertension to monitor blood pressure, and people with cancer to monitor their white blood cell counts. These innovations allow hospitals to remain the central hub of care if necessary while becoming a last resort rather than a first point of entry. Other innovations relating to improved system design and better information systems also have the potential to improve care and, assuming that the systems are not too expensive, contain costs at the same time. Many of these models involve giving explicit responsibility for care coordination to someone to ensure that the necessary services are provided.

A related set of options, also noted earlier, deals with who delivers care. There have been efforts around labour substitution to try to ensure that higher cost workers are used only for activities that cannot be done by others. The extent to which this can save money is clearly related to the nature of the funding model (e.g., if the payer will only reimburse for services provided by a physician, then we have little reason to have those services provided by other practitioners.) However, considerable experiments with changing how (and by whom) care is delivered have taken place, including replacing doctors with nurses (or nurse practitioners) or midwives, replacing RNs with less trained registered practical nurses, replacing nurses with personal support workers, replacing PSWs with unpaid caregivers (volunteers or family members), encouraging self-care, and so on. Other potential reforms, particularly as technology improves, may incorporate contracting out services to lower cost providers. This has been less pronounced in health care than in other services, but if the licensure requirements can be dealt with, can we foresee a day when telehealth lets us use foreign care providers to staff call centres to treat us online? Would this be a good idea?

Improve Efficiency

The last reform suggestion in the Introduction was to become more efficient and get better value for money. Clearly, these reform suggestions do not stand alone; many of the possible reforms we have already discussed have the potential to improve efficiency. A number of policy levers suggest themselves.

An obvious starting point is to reduce waste. Defining waste is tricky, but it usually means spending that could be eliminated without harming those receiving care or reducing their quality of care. There are a number of potential targets. Some obvious low-hanging fruit would also improve quality of care. As noted earlier, the patient safety movement is focusing on such things as avoiding preventable injuries, such as by making sure people do not get infectious diseases while in hospitals or receive the wrong medications. Another easy fix is to avoid fraud and abuse, such as by not paying for services that were not delivered. This may involve implementing various audit trails (while ensuring that the administrative costs of these mechanisms do not exceed the potential savings).

Despite frequent discussion of waste, it is important to note that Canada's system already appears to be relatively efficient. Woolhandler and Himmelstein accessed 1999 data (as available) and analysed the costs of insurers, employers, doctors, hospitals, nursing homes, and home care agencies in the United States and Canada. Their computations suggested that administration consumed 31% of US spending, as compared with 16.7% for Canada. Looking only at the single-payer component of health expenditures, they estimated that Canada was spending 1.3% on administration, as compared with 3.6% for the US publicly funded program (Medicare) and 11.7% for overhead for the US private insurers. Their conclusion, which drew considerable attention, was that if the United States could get their administrative spending to the same level as Canada, there would be enough savings to extend full coverage to the entire US population.[17] For example, a physician would not have to pay staff to see which of many possible insurance plans their patient belonged to and what forms they needed to fill out, since they would usually have only one set of forms to complete. Another study by this team comparing hospital administrative costs in eight countries (Canada, England, Scotland, Wales, France, Germany, the Netherlands, and the United States) found that Canada and Scotland had by far the lowest administrative costs.[18]

Another obvious target for improving efficiency, which we have referred to frequently in this book, is appropriateness; it is usually advisable not to spend money to purchase services that are not likely to produce better health outcomes for that person. Again, we must confront issues about how good the evidence needs to be before we decide something is worth doing. Another target is inefficiencies and looking for ways to produce the same outcomes for less cost. However, we must ensure that the people who provide the care are paid fairly (where "fairly" is clearly going to be open to dispute).

Moving to the bulk of health expenditures, we can also identify possible strategies. Health economists have suggested that health care costs can be broken down as follows: if each item purchased has a cost, the total spending on that item is the number purchased (often called the *volume of services*) times the cost, which would make the total spending for health care the sum of the cost times the volume for each of the entire set of items that are being purchased. This in turn points to three areas for cost control. One is the cost of each item. The second is the volume. The third is the mix of items.

Cost would appear to be the simplest of these. Presumably, payers could try to negotiate better prices. They may work with other organizations and use joint purchasing. They may seek efficiencies in how they deliver care, including controlling wages and benefits, using labour substitution (e.g., many nursing homes have replaced some of their nurses with PSWs), centralizing back office functions, and the like. Since the least expensive worker is one you don't have to pay, there is also a trend to try to get patients to manage their own care or rely on their friends and family to help them. There may also be considerable scope for efficiencies through service integration, as noted above. However, we must ensure that the people providing these services receive fair wages, so there are likely to be limits in potential savings once the obvious inefficiencies are addressed.

Volume and item mix tend to work together, particularly if we can substitute treatments. For example, if someone could be treated by different medications, changing what drug was prescribed would reduce the volume of product A while increasing the volume of product B. Similarly, we might substitute surgical treatment with watch and wait. Efforts to avoid unnecessary or inappropriate treatment can thus affect volume and the mix of items, and in the best case also improve outcomes, if other lower cost services would indeed be appropriate for those clients.

Conclusion

How should we fix health care? What is broken? Unfortunately, there is no single answer. Health care tends to be individual; people need the right care, at the right time, at the right place, at the right price. Fortunately, most of the time, that is what we get, particularly when we are really sick. But that depends heavily on who we are, where we live, what health problems we have, and which providers we are seeing. This implies that most reforms will tend to be incremental. Moving items around on an organizational chart may seem momentarily satisfying but is unlikely to make a major impact on performance. We conclude that although there is no obvious one-size-fits-all reform, a number of smaller reforms are likely to be helpful. These include paying more attention to how to keep people healthier, focusing on appropriateness, and continuing to work to improve service integration and quality of care. More attention to what should be considered an insured service might also help; suggestions that this should be based on medical necessity rather than only on where care is delivered and by whom could be helpful. The frequent suggestions to expand what is covered, with particular attention to pharmacare, home care, and mental health, seem highly promising.

The final conclusion? Things are pretty good. But they could be better. With luck and dedicated payers, regulators, providers, patients, and caregivers, they will be.

Notes

Introduction

1 Raisa B. Deber and Catherine L. Mah, *Case Studies in Canadian Health Policy and Management*, 2nd ed. (Toronto, ON: University of Toronto Press, 2014).

1 Defining Our Terms: What Is Health Policy? What Is Health?

1 W.I. Jenkins, *Policy Analysis: A Political and Organizational Perspective* (London, UK: M. Robertson, 1978).
2 Peter Bachrach and Morton S. Baratz, "Decisions and Nondecisions: An Analytical Framework," *American Political Science Review* 57, no. 3 (1963): 632–42, doi:10.2307/1952568.
3 Aaron Wildavsky, *Speaking Truth to Power: The Art and Craft of Policy Analysis*, 2nd ed. (Boston, MA: Little Brown and Company, 1979).
4 Deborah A. Stone, *Policy Paradox: The Art of Political Decision Making*, 3rd ed. (New York, NY: Norton, 2011).
5 G. Bruce Doern and Richard W. Phidd, *Canadian Public Policy: Ideas, Structure, Process*, 2nd ed. (Toronto, ON: Nelson Canada, 1992).
6 World Health Organization, *Preamble to the Constitution of the World Health Organization as Adopted by the International Health Conference* (Geneva, Switzerland: WHO, 1948), accessed March 15, 2017, http://www.who.int/about/mission/en/.
7 Marc Lalonde, *A New Perspective on the Health of Canadians: A Working Document* (Ottawa, ON: Minister of Supply and Services Canada, 1974), accessed March 15, 2017, http://www.phac-aspc.gc.ca/ph-sp/pdf/perspect-eng.pdf.

8 Public Health Agency of Canada, *What Determines Health?* (Ottawa, ON: Government of Canada, 2011), accessed March 15, 2017, http://www .phac-aspc.gc.ca/ph-sp/determinants/index-eng.php.

9 Juha Mikkonen and Dennis Raphael, *Social Determinants of Health: The Canadian Facts* (Toronto, ON: York University School of Health Policy and Management, 2010), accessed March 15, 2017, http://www.the canadianfacts.org/The_Canadian_Facts.pdf; Public Health Agency of Canada, *Public Health Topics: Social Determinants of Health* (Ottawa, ON: Government of Canada, 2016), accessed March 15, 2017, http://cbpp-pcpe .phac-aspc.gc.ca/public-health-topics/social-determinants-of-health/.

10 World Health Organization, *Social Determinants of Health* (Geneva, Switzerland: WHO, 2016), accessed March 15, 2017, http://www.who.int /social_determinants/en/.

11 John M. Last, *A Dictionary of Epidemiology*, 2nd ed. (New York, NY: Oxford University Press, 1988).

12 World Health Organization, *Ottawa Charter for Health Promotion, 1986* (Ottawa, ON: WHO, 1986), accessed March 15, 2017, http://www.phac -aspc.gc.ca/ph-sp/docs/charter-chartre/index-eng.php.

13 Public Health Agency of Canada, *What Is the Population Health Approach?* (Ottawa, ON: Government of Canada, 2012), accessed March 15, 2017, http://www.phac-aspc.gc.ca/ph-sp/approach-approche/index-eng.php.

14 Standing Senate Committee on Social Affairs Science and Technology, *A Healthy, Productive Canada: A Determinant of Health Approach*. Final report of Senate Subcommittee on Population Health (Ottawa, ON: Senate, 2009), accessed March 15, 2017, https://sencanada.ca/content /sen/Committee/402/popu/rep/rephealth1jun09-e.pdf.

2   What Is Health Care?

1 Robert G. Evans, *Strained Mercy: The Economics of Canadian Health Care* (Toronto, ON: Butterworths & Co., 1984).

2 Raisa Deber, "Access without Appropriateness: Chicken Little in Charge?" *Healthcare Policy* 4, no. 1 (2008): 23–9, https://www.ncbi.nlm.nih.gov /pmc/articles/PMC2645207/.

3 Barbara Starfield, "Toward International Primary Care Reform," *Canadian Medical Association Journal* 180, no. 11 (2009): 1091–2, http://www .cmaj.ca/cgi/content/full/180/11/1091.

4 Mireille Dumont-Lemasson, Carol Donovan, and Maggie Wylie, *Provincial and Territorial Home Care Programs: A Synthesis for Canada* (Ottawa, ON: Health Canada, 1999), accessed March 15, 2017, http://www.hc-sc.gc.ca /hcs-sss/pubs/home-domicile/1999-pt-synthes/index-eng.php.

5 Peggy Leatt, George H. Pink, and Michael Guerriere, "Towards a Canadian
   Model of Integrated Healthcare," *Healthcare Papers* 1, no. 2 (2000):
   13–35, http://www.longwoods.com/content/17216.
6 Eliot Freidson, *Professionalism, the Third Logic* (Chicago, IL: University of
   Chicago Press, 2001).
7 Canadian Association of Naturopathic Doctors, *Common questions:
   Education and regulation* (Toronto, ON: CAND, 2016), accessed March 15,
   2017, http://www.cand.ca/common-questions-education-and-regulation/.
8 A. Paul Williams, Allie Peckham, Kerry Kuluski, Janet Lum, Natalie
   Warrick, Karen Spalding, Tommy Tam, Cindy Bruce-Barrett, Marta
   Grasic, and Jennifer Im, "Caring for Caregivers: Challenging the Assump-
   tions," *HealthcarePapers* 15, no. 1 (2015): 8–21, http://www.longwoods
   .com/content/24401; A. Paul Williams, Janet Lum, Frances Morton-Chang,
   Kerry Kuluski, Allie Peckham, Natalie Warrick, and Alvin Ying, *Integrating
   Long-Term Care into a Community-Based Continuum: Shifting from "Beds"
   to "Places"* (Toronto, ON: Institute for Research on Public Policy, 2016),
   accessed March 15, 2017, http://irpp.org/wp-content/uploads/2016/02
   /study-no59.pdf.
9 Mohamad Alameddine, Audrey Laporte, Andrea Baumann, Linda
   O'Brien-Pallas, Barbara Mildon, and Raisa Deber, "'Stickiness' and
   'Inflow' as Proxy Measures of the Relative Attractiveness of Various
   Sub-Sectors of Nursing Employment," *Social Science & Medicine* 63, no. 9
   (2006): 2310–19, https://www.ncbi.nlm.nih.gov/pubmed/16781038.
10 An extensive list of links to material on health human resources is
   available from the Canadian Health Human Resources Research Network,
   http://www.hhr-rhs.ca/.
11 Jacques Gallant, "Ontario Midwives Allege Gender-Based Pay Gap,
   Compared to Doctors," *Toronto Star*, May 31, 2016, accessed March 15,
   2017, https://www.thestar.com/news/gta/2016/05/31/ontario-midwives
   -allege-gender-based-pay-gap-compared-to-doctors.html.

3 How Is Health Care Paid For and Delivered?

1 Jeremiah Hurley, *Health Economics* (Whitby, ON: McGraw-Hill Ryerson,
   2010).
2 Ontario Ministry of Health and Long-Term Care, *Get Coverage for
   Prescription Drugs* (Toronto, ON: Queen's Printer for Ontario, 2016),
   accessed March 15, 2017, https://www.ontario.ca/page/get-coverage
   -prescription-drugs.
3 Raisa B. Deber, "Delivering Health Care Services: Public, Not-for-Profit,
   or Private?" in *The Fiscal Sustainability of Health Care in Canada:*

Romanow Papers, Volume 1, ed. Gregory P. Marchildon, Tom McIntosh, and Pierre-Gerlier Forest (Toronto, ON: University of Toronto Press, 2004), 233–96; Robert G. Evans, *Strained Mercy: The Economics of Canadian Health Care* (Toronto, ON: Butterworths & Co., 1984).

4 Organisation for Economic Co-operation and Development, *About: What We Do and How* (Paris, France: OECD, 2016) [cited 2017], accessed March 15, 2017, http://www.oecd.org/about/whatwedoandhow/.

5 Owen Adams and Sharon Vanin, "Funding Long-Term Care in Canada: Issues and Options," *HealthcarePapers* 15, no. 4 (2016): 7–19, http://www.longwoods.com/content/24583; Raisa B. Deber and A. Laporte, "Funding Long-Term Care in Canada: Who Is Responsible for What?" *HealthcarePapers* 15, no. 4 (2016): 36–40. Available from http://www.longwoods.com/content/24587.

6 Deber, "Delivering Health Care Services" in *The Fiscal Sustainability of Health Care in Canada*; Gregory P. Marchildon, *Canada: Health System Review* (Copenhagen, Denmark: European Observatory on Health Systems and Policies, 2013), accessed March 15, 2017, http://www.euro.who.int/__data/assets/pdf_file/0011/181955/e96759.pdf; Raisa Deber, "Canada," in *Cost Containment and Efficiency in National Health Systems: A Global Comparison*, ed. John Rapoport, Philip Jacobs, and Egon Jonsson (Weinheim, Germany: Wiley-VCH Verlag GmbH & Co., 2009), 15–39.

7 Elizabeth Docteur and Howard Oxley, *Health-Care Systems: Lessons from the Reform Experience* (Paris, France: OECD Publishing, 2003), accessed March 15, 2017, http://www.oecd-ilibrary.org/social-issues-migration-health/health-care-systems_865047648066; Raisa Deber and Kenneth C.K. Lam, *Medical Savings Accounts in Financing Healthcare*, Canadian Health Services Research Foundation (CHSRF) Reports on Financing Models: Paper 3 (Ottawa, ON: CHSRF, 2011), accessed March 15, 2017, http://www.cfhi-fcass.ca/sf-docs/default-source/commissioned-research-reports/RAISA3-MedicalSAcc_EN.pdf?sfvrsn=0; Raisa Deber and Kenneth C.K. Lam, *Experience with Medical Savings Accounts in Selected Jurisdictions*, CHSRF Series of Reports on Financing Models: Paper 4 (Ottawa, ON: CHSRF, 2011), accessed March 15, 2017, http://www.cfhi-fcass.ca/sf-docs/default-source/commissioned-research-reports/RAISA4_Experience_in_MSA_EN.pdf?sfvrsn=0; Francesca Colombo and Nicole Tapay, *Private Health Insurance in OECD Countries: The Benefits and Costs for Individuals and Health Systems*, OECD Health Working Papers, No. 15 (Paris, France: OECD Health, 2004), accessed March 15, 2017, https://www.oecd.org/els/health-systems/33698043.pdf; Sara Allin, Mark Stabile

and Carolyn Hughes Tuohy, *Financing Models for Non-Canada Health Act Services in Canada: Lessons from Local and International Experiences with Social Insurance*, CHSRF Series of Reports on Financing Models: Paper 2 (Ottawa, ON: CHSRF, 2010), accessed March 15, 2017, http://www .cfhi-fcass.ca/sf-docs/default-source/commissioned-research-reports /CHSRF_4FinancingModels_En-final2.pdf?sfvrsn=0.

8 Deber, "Delivering Health Care Services," in *The Fiscal Sustainability of Health Care in Canada*.

9 Alexander S. Preker, April Harding, and Phyllida Travis, "'Make or Buy' Decisions in the Production of Health Care Goods and Services: New Insights from Institutional Economics and Organizational Theory," *Bulletin of the World Health Organization* 78, no. 6 (2000): 779–89, accessed March 15, 2017, http://www.who.int/bulletin/archives/78(6)779 .pdf.

10 Raisa Deber, Marcus J. Hollander, and Philip Jacobs, "Models of Funding and Reimbursement in Health Care: A Conceptual Framework," *Canadian Public Administration* 51, no. 3 (2008): 381–405, http://onlinelibrary .wiley.com/doi/10.1111/j.1754-7121.2008.00030.x/full.

11 Pierre Thomas Leger, "Physician Payment Mechanisms," in *Financing Health Care: New Ideas for a Changing Society*, ed. Mingshan Lu and Egon Jonsson (Weinheim, Germany: Wiley-VCH Verlag GmbH & Co, KGaA, 2008), 149–76.

12 Committee on Quality of Health Care in America and Institute of Medicine, *Crossing the Quality Chasm: A New Health System for the 21st Century* (Washington, DC: National Academy Press, 2001).

13 Raisa B. Deber, Kenneth C.K. Lam, and Leslie L. Roos, "Four Flavours of Health Expenditures: A Discussion of the Potential Implications of the Distribution of Health Expenditures for Financing Health Care," *Canadian Public Policy* 40, no. 4 (2014): 353–63, doi:10.3138/cpp.2014-018.

4 How Does Canada Do It?

1 *Constitution Act, 1867* (UK), 30 & 31 Vict, c 3, reprinted in RSC 1985, Appendix II, No 5; and *Constitution Act, 1982*, being Schedule B to the Canada Act 1982 (UK), 1982, c 11. accessed March 15, 2017, http:// laws-lois.justice.gc.ca/eng/Const/FullText.html.

2 Christopher W. McDougall, David Kirsch, Brian Schwartz, and Raisa Deber, "Looking for Trouble: Developing and Implementing a National Network for Infectious Disease Surveillance in Canada," in *Case Studies*

in Canadian Health Policy and Management, 2nd ed., ed. Raisa B. Deber and Catherine L. Mah (Toronto, ON: University of Toronto Press, 2014), 179–205.

3 Department of Finance Canada, *Federal Support to Provinces and Territories* (Ottawa, ON: Government of Canada, 2016), accessed March 15, 2017, http://www.fin.gc.ca/access/fedprov-eng.asp#Major.

4 Marchildon, *Canada: Health System Review*; Malcolm G. Taylor, *Health Insurance and Canadian Public Policy. The Seven Decisions That Created the Canadian Health Insurance System and Their Outcomes*, 2nd ed. (Kingston, ON: McGill-Queen's University Press, 1987).

5 C. Stuart Houston, *Hospital Services Plan* (Regina, SK: University of Regina and Canadian Plains Research Center, 2005), accessed March 15, 2017, http://esask.uregina.ca/entry/hospital_services_plan.html.

6 Walter O. Spitzer, David L. Sackett, John C. Sibley, Robin S. Roberts, Michael Gent, Dorothy J. Kergin, Brenda C. Hackett, and Anthony Olynich, "The Burlington Randomized Trial of the Nurse Practitioner," *New England Journal of Medicine* 290, no. 5 (1974): 251–6.

7 Department of Finance Canada, *Federal Investments in Health Care* (Ottawa, ON: Government of Canada, 2012), accessed March 15, 2017, https://www.fin.gc.ca/fedprov/fihc-ifass-eng.asp.

8 Colleen M. Flood and Sujit Choudhry, "Strengthening the Foundations: Modernizing the Canada Health Act," in *The Governance of Health Care in Canada: Romanow Papers, Volume 3*, ed. Tom McIntosh, Pierre-Gerlier Forest, and Gregory P. Marchildon (Toronto, ON: University of Toronto Press, 2004), 346–87; Colleen M. Flood, Kent Roach, and Lorne Sossin, *Access to Care, Access to Justice: The Legal Debate over Private Health Insurance in Canada* (Toronto, ON: University of Toronto Press, 2005); Odette Madore, *The Canada Health Act: Overview and Options*, Current Issue Review 94-4E (Ottawa, ON: Library of Parliament, 2005), accessed March 15, 2017, https://lop.parl.ca/content/lop/ResearchPublications /944-e.htm.

9 Health Canada, *Health Care System: Reports and Publications – Canada Health Act Annual Reports* (Ottawa, ON: Government of Canada, 2016), accessed March 15, 2017, http://www.hc-sc.gc.ca/hcs-sss/pubs/cha-lcs /index-eng.php.

10 Catherine A. Charles, Jonathan Lomas, and Mita Giacomini, "Medical Necessity in Canadian Health Policy: Four Meanings and ... A Funeral?" *Milbank Quarterly* 75, no. 3 (1997): 365–94, https://www.ncbi.nlm.nih .gov/pubmed/9290634.

11 *Canada Health Act,* RSC, 1985, c. C-6, accessed March 15, 2017, http://laws-lois.justice.gc.ca/eng/acts/C-6/.

12 Madore, *The Canada Health Act: Overview and Options.*

13 Commission on the Future of Health Care in Canada, *Building on Values: The Future of Health Care in Canada, Final Report* (Ottawa, ON: Queen's Printer, 2002), accessed March 15, 2017, http://publications.gc.ca/collections/Collection/CP32-85-2002E.pdf; Gregory P. Marchildon, Tom McIntosh, and Pierre-Gerlier Forest, *The Fiscal Sustainability of Health Care in Canada: Romanow Papers, Volume 1* (Toronto, ON: University of Toronto Press, 2004); Pierre-Gerlier Forest, Gregory P. Marchildon, and Tom McIntosh, *Changing Health Care in Canada: Romanow Papers, Volume 2* (Toronto, ON: University of Toronto Press, 2004); Tom McIntosh, Pierre-Gerlier Forest, and Gregory P. Marchildon, *The Governance of Health Care in Canada: Romanow Papers, Volume 3* (Toronto, ON: University of Toronto Press, 2004).

14 Standing Senate Committee on Social Affairs Science and Technology, *The Health of Canadians – The Federal Role. Volume Six: Recommendations for Reform* (Ottawa, ON: Parliament of Canada, 2002), accessed March 15, 2017, https://sencanada.ca/content/sen/committee/372/soci/rep/repoct02vol6-e.htm.

15 Deber, "Delivering Health Care Services," in *The Fiscal Sustainability of Health Care in Canada.*

16 *Chaoulli v. Quebec (Attorney General),* [2005] 1 SCR 791, 2005 SCC 35. Available from: https://scc-csc.lexum.com/scc-csc/scc-csc/en/item/2237/index.do; Odette Madore, *Duplicate Private Health Care Insurance: Potential Implications for Quebec and Canada* (Ottawa, ON: Library of Parliament, 2006), accessed March 15, 2017, https://lop.parl.ca/content/lop/ResearchPublications/prb0571-e.htm.

17 Richard B. Saltman, Vaida Bankauskaite, and Karsten Vrangbaek, *Decentralization in Health Care* (Berkshire, UK: Open University Press, 2007); Juha Kinnunen, Kirill Danishevski, Raisa B. Deber, and Theodore H. Tulchinsky, "Effects of Decentralization on Clinical Dimensions of Health Systems," in *Decentralization in Health Care,* ed. Richard B. Saltman, Vaida Bankauskaite, and Karsten Vrangbaek (Berkshire, UK: Open University Press, 2007), 167–88; Gregory P. Marchildon, "Health Care," in *The Oxford Handbook of Canadian Politics,* ed. John C. Courtney, David E. Smith (Oxford, UK: Oxford University Press, 2010), 111–30.

18 Ministry of Health and Long-Term Care, *Local Health Integration Networks (LHINs): Building a True System* (Toronto, ON: Government of

Ontario, 2004), accessed March 15, 2017, http://www.ontla.on.ca/library /repository/ser/247449/2006/2006no21.pdf.

19 Ministry of Health and Long-Term Care, *About the Ministry* (Toronto, ON: Government of Ontario, 2017), accessed March 15, 2017, http://www .health.gov.on.ca/en/common/ministry/default.aspx.

20 Government of Ontario, *Patients First: A Roadmap to Strengthen Home and Community Care* (Toronto, Ontario: Government of Ontario, 2015), accessed March 15, 2017, http://www.health.gov.on.ca/en/public /programs/ccac/roadmap.pdf.

21 Canadian Institute for Health Information, *About CIHI* (Ottawa, ON: CIHI, 2016), accessed March 15, 2017, https://www.cihi.ca/en/about-cihi. The CIHI website can be consulted for up-to-date information; a wide variety of useful reports and data files are also available for download. See the CIHI homepage at https://www.cihi.ca/en.

22 Canadian Institute for Health Information, *National Health Expenditure Trends, 1975 to 2015* (Ottawa, ON: CIHI, 2015), accessed March 15, 2017, https://www.cihi.ca/sites/default/files/document/nhex_trends_narrative_ report_2015_en.pdf.

23 Government of Canada, *News Release: Government of Canada Partners with Provinces and Territories to Lower Cost of Pharmaceuticals* (Ottawa, ON: Health Canada, January 19, 2016), accessed March 15, 2017, http:// news.gc.ca/web/article-en.do?nid=1028339.

24 Steven G. Morgan, Marc-André Gagnon, Barbara Mintzes, and Joel Lexchin, "A Better Prescription: Advice for a National Strategy on Pharma- ceutical Policy in Canada," *Healthcare Policy* 12, no. 1 (2016): 18–36, http://www.longwoods.com/content/24637.

25 Raisa Deber and Kenneth C.K. Lam, "Handling the High Spenders: Implications of the Distribution of Health Expenditures for Financing Health Care," APSA 2009 Toronto meeting paper, 2009, accessed March 15, 2017, https://papers.ssrn.com/Sol3/papers.cfm?abstract_ id=1450788.

5   Health Care in Canada: International Comparisons

1 European Observatory on Health Care Systems and Policies. *Health System Reviews (HiT Series)* (2017), accessed March 16, 2017, http://www .euro.who.int/en/about-us/partners/observatory/publications/health -system-reviews-hits.

2 Elias Mossialos, Martin Wenzl, Robin Osborn, and Dana Sarnak, eds., *International Profiles of Health Care Systems, 2015: Australia, Canada,*

China, Denmark, England, France, Germany, India, Israel, Italy, Japan, The Netherlands, New Zealand, Norway, Singapore, Sweden, Switzerland, and the United States (New York, NY: Commonwealth Fund, 2016), accessed March 16, 2017, http://www.commonwealthfund.org/~/media/files/publications/fund-report/2016/jan/1857_mossialos_intl_profiles_2015_v7.pdf?la=en.

3 Evidence Network, *International Health Systems* (2016), accessed March 16, 2017, http://evidencenetwork.ca/international-health-systems.

4 World Health Organization, *Health Topics: Health Systems* (Geneva, Switzerland: WHO, 2017), accessed March 16, 2017, http://www.who.int/topics/health_systems/en/.

5 Henry E. Sigerist, "From Bismarck to Beveridge: Developments and Trends in Social Security Legislation," *Journal of Public Health Policy* 20, no. 4 (1999): 474–96.

6 David U. Himmelstein, Elizabeth Warren, Deborah Thorne, and Steffie Woolhandler, "Illness and Injury as Contributors to Bankruptcy," *Health Affairs*. Published online February 2, 2005: 63–73, http://content.healthaffairs.org/content/early/2005/02/02/hlthaff.w5.63.full.pdf.

7 World Health Organization, *The World Health Report 2000: Health Systems: Improving Performance* (Geneva, Switzerland: WHO, 2000), accessed March 16, 2017, http://www.who.int/whr/2000/en/.

8 Raisa Deber, "Why Did the World Health Organization Rate Canada's Health System as 30th? Some Thoughts on League Tables," *Healthcare Quarterly* 7, no. 2 (2003): 2–7, http://www.longwoods.com/content/17238.

9 The data being used in Table 5.1 come from Organisation for Economic Co-operation and Development, *OECD Health Statistics 2016* (Paris, France: OECD, 2016), accessed March 16, 2017, http://www.oecd.org/health/health-data.htm. I am using the most recent data, which it describes as "2015 or nearest year," or as "2014 or nearest year" depending on how much missing data they had. Table 5.1 includes the year they specify for each metric, recognizing that in some cases the numbers used came from earlier years. Note that the OECD has also made some slight changes in how it defines particular variables, which means that the specific numbers in the dataset it published in 2016 are not always completely comparable with some of the numbers published for previous years, although the differences are not large. Since Latvia joined the EU in 2016, the rankings may also have changed, since the tables reflect 35 rather than 34 countries.

10 Organisation for Economic Co-operation and Development, *Purchasing Power Parities – Frequently Asked Questions (FAQs)* (Paris, France: OECD,

2016), accessed March 16, 2017, http://www.oecd.org/std/prices-ppp
/purchasingpowerparities-frequentlyaskedquestionsfaqs.htm.

11 *OECD Health Statistics 2016*, accessed March 16, 2017, http://www.oecd.
org/health/health-data.htm.

12 Karen Davis, Kristof Stremikis, David Squires, and Cathy Schoen, *Mirror,
Mirror on the Wall: How the Performance of the US Health Care System
Compares Internationally* (Washington, DC: Commonwealth Fund, 2014),
accessed March 16, 2017, http://www.commonwealthfund.org/~/media
/files/publications/fund-report/2014/jun/1755_davis_mirror_mirror_2014.
pdf.

13 Davis, Stremikis, Squires, and Schoen, *Mirror, Mirror.*

14 Health Council of Canada, *Where You Live Matters: Canadian Views on
Health Care Quality* (Toronto, ON: Health Council of Canada, 2014),
accessed March 16, 2017, http://www.healthcouncilcanada.ca/content_lm
.php?mnu=2&mnu1=48&mnu2=30&mnu3=56.

15 Statistics Canada, *Access to a Regular Medical Doctor, 2014* (Ottawa, ON:
2014), accessed March 16, 2017, http://www.statcan.gc.ca/pub/82-625-x
/2015001/article/14177-eng.htm.

16 Mark Britnell, *In Search of the Perfect Health System* (London, UK:
Palgrave, 2015).

17 Gordon H. Guyatt, P.J. Devereaux, Joel Lexchin, Samuel B. Stone, Armine
Yalnizyan, David Himmelstein, Steffie Woolhandler, et al., "A Systematic
Review of Studies Comparing Health Outcomes in Canada and the United
States," *Open Medicine* 1, no. 1 (2007): E27–E36; Organisation for
Economic Co-operation and Development, *Health at a Glance 2015: How
Does Canada Compare?* (Paris, France: OECD, 2015), accessed March 16,
2017, https://www.oecd.org/canada/Health-at-a-Glance-2015-Key
-Findings-CANADA.pdf.

6 How Should We Decide What Is Worth Paying For?

1 Tony Culyer, *The Humble Economist: Tony Culyer on Health, Health Care
and Social Decision Making*, Richard Cookson, Clare Brayshaw, eds. (York,
UK: York Publishing Services, Ltd., 2012).

2 Marthe R. Gold, Joanna E. Siegel, Louise B. Russell, and Milton C.
Weinstein, *Cost-Effectiveness in Health and Medicine* (New York, NY:
Oxford University Press, 1996); Michael F. Drummond, Mark J. Sculpher,
George W. Torrance, Bernard O'Brien, and Greg Stoddart, *Methods for the
Economic Evaluation of Health Care Programmes*, 3rd ed. (Toronto, ON:
Oxford University Press, 2005).

3 Amos Tversky and Daniel Kahneman, "The Framing of Decisions and the
   Psychology of Choice," *Science* 211, no. 4481 (1981): 453–8, doi:10.1126
   /science.7455683..
4 Raisa B. Deber, "Translating Technology Assessment into Policy:
   Conceptual Issues and Tough Choices," *International Journal of Technology Assessment in Health Care* 8, no. 1 (1992): 131–7.
5 Tito Fojo and Christine Grady, "How Much Is Life Worth: Cetuximab,
   Non-small Cell Lung Cancer, and the $440 billion question," *Journal of
   the National Cancer Institute* 101, no. 15 (2009): 1044–8, doi:10.1093
   /jnci/djp177.
6 Steve Buist, "New Cancer Drugs Raise Hope for Patients, but Carry Steep
   Costs," *Toronto Star*, February 29, 2016, accessed March 16, 2017, https://
   www.thestar.com/news/insight/2016/02/28/medical-advances-to
   -extend-cancer-survival-rates-outpacing-our-ability-to-pay-for
   -treatments.html.
7 Andrew Dillon, *Carrying NICE over the Threshold – Blog* (London, England: National Institute for Health and Clinical Excellence, 2015),
   accessed March 16, 2017, https://www.nice.org.uk/news/blog/carrying
   -nice-over-the-threshold.
8 Jeffrey Peppercorn, S. Yousuf Zafar, Kevin Houck, Peter Ubel, and Neal J.
   Meropol, "Does Comparative Effectiveness Research Promote Rationing
   of Cancer Care?" *The Lancet Oncology* 15, no. 3 (2014): e132–e138. Epub
   February 14, 2014, accessed March 16, 2017, doi:10.1016/S1470-2045
   (13)70597-7.
9 Peter J. Neumann and Milton C. Weinstein, "Legislating against Use of
   Cost-Effectiveness Information," *New England Journal of Medicine* 363,
   no. 13 (2010): 1495–7. doi:10.1056/NEJMp1007168.
10 Raisa Deber, "Access without Appropriateness: Chicken Little in Charge?"
   Healthcare Policy 4, no. 1 (2008): 23–9, https://www.ncbi.nlm.nih.gov
   /pmc/articles/PMC2645207/.
11 Choosing Wisely Canada, *Home Page* (Toronto, ON: 2017), accessed
   March 16, 2017, http://www.choosingwiselycanada.org/.
12 Deber and Mah, *Case Studies in Canadian Health Policy and Management*.
13 Raisa Deber, "Access without Appropriateness: Chicken Little in Charge?".
14 World Health Organization, *Appropriateness in Health Care Services:
   Report on a WHO Workshop, Koblenz, Germany (23–25 March 2000)*
   (Copenhagen, Denmark: WHO, 2000), accessed March 16, 2017, http://
   www.euro.who.int/__data/assets/pdf_file/0011/119936/E70446.pdf.
15 T.L. Beauchamp and J.F. Childress, *Principles of Biomedical Ethics*, 5th ed.
   (New York, NY: Oxford University Press, 2001).

16 Stone, *Policy Paradox: The Art of Political Decision Making.*
17 Norman Daniels, "Accountability for Reasonableness," *British Medical Journal* 321, no. 7272 (2000): 1300–1, https://www.ncbi.nlm.nih.gov/pmc/articles/PMC1119050/; Norman Daniels and James Sabin, "The Ethics of Accountability in Managed Care Reform," *Health Affairs* 17, no. 5 (1998): 50–64; Douglas K. Martin, Mita Giacomini, and Peter Singer, "Fairness, Accountability for Reasonableness, and the Views of Priority Setting Decision-Makers," *Health Policy* 61, no. 3 (2002): 279–90.
18 Jennifer Gibson, Douglas Martin, and Peter Singer, "Evidence, Economics and Ethics: Resource Allocation in Health Service Organizations," *Healthcare Quarterly* 8, no. 2 (2005): 50–9.
19 Elmer Eric Schattschneider, *The Semisovereign People: A Realist's View of Democracy in America*, 3rd ed. (New York, NY: Holt, Rinehart and Winston, 1975).
20 David Kriebel and Joel Tickner, "The Precautionary Principle and Public health: Reenergizing Public Health through Precaution," *American Journal of Public Health* 91, no. 9 (2001): 1351–5, http://ajph.aphapublications.org/doi/pdf/10.2105/AJPH.91.9.1351.
21 Erica Weir, Richard Schabas, Kumanan Wilson, and Chris Mackie, "A Canadian Framework for Applying the Precautionary Principle to Public Health Issues," *Canadian Journal of Public Health* 101, no. 5 (2010): 396–8, http://journal.cpha.ca/index.php/cjph/article/viewArticle/2635.
22 Guido Calabresi and Philip Bobbit, *Tragic Choices: The Conflicts Society Confronts in the Allocation of Tragically Scarce Resources* (New York, NY: W.W. Norton & Company, 1978).
23 Norman Daniels, "Four Unsolved Rationing Problems: A Challenge," *Hastings Centre Report* 24, no. 4 (1994): 27–9.
24 Morgan, Gagnon, Mintzes, and Lexchin, "A Better Prescription."
25 André Picard, "With Supplements, Never Assume 'Natural' Means Safe," *Globe and Mail,* May 31, 2016, accessed March 16, 2017, http://www.theglobeandmail.com/opinion/with-supplements-never-assume-natural-means-safe/article30212467/.
26 Canadian Agency for Drugs and Technologies in Health, *About CADTH* (Ottawa, ON: CADTH, 2017), accessed March 16, 2017, https://www.cadth.ca/about-cadth.
27 Patricia M. Baranek, Raisa Deber, and A. Paul Williams, *Almost Home: Reforming Home and Community Care in Ontario* (Toronto, ON: University of Toronto Press, 2004).
28 Committee on Quality of Health Care in America and Institute of Medicine, *Crossing the Quality Chasm: A New Health System for the 21st Century.*

29 CBC News, "Alberta Parents Convicted in Toddler's Meningitis Death,"
    April 26, 2016, accessed March 16, 2017, http://www.cbc.ca/news/canada
    /calgary/meningitis-trial-verdict-1.3552941.
30 Raisa B. Deber, Nancy Kraetschmer, and Jane Irvine, "What Role Do
    Patients Wish to Play in Treatment Decision Making?" *Archives of
    Internal Medicine* 156, no. 13 (1996): 1414–20; Nancy Kraetschmer,
    Natasha Sharpe, Sara Urowitz, and Raisa B. Deber, "How Does Trust
    Affect Patient Preferences for Participation in Decision Making?" *Health
    Expectations* 7, no. 4 (2004): 317–26; Raisa B. Deber, Nancy Kraetschmer,
    Sara Urowitz, and Natasha Sharpe, "Do People Want to be Autonomous
    Patients? Preferred Roles in Treatment Decision-Making in Several
    Patient Populations," *Health Expectations* 10, no. 3 (2007): 248–58.
31 France Légaré and Holly O. Witteman, "Shared Decision Making:
    Examining Key Elements and Barriers to Adoption into Routine Clinical
    Practice," *Health Affairs* 32, no. 2 (2013): 276–84, https://www.ncbi.nlm
    .nih.gov/pubmed/23381520; Michael J. Barry and Susan Edgman-Levitan,
    "Shared Decision Making – The Pinnacle of Patient-Centered Care,"
    New England Journal of Medicine 366, no. 9 (2012): 780–1.

7 Pressing Issues

1 Danielle Martin, *Better Now: Six Big Ideas to Improve Health Care for All
   Canadians*, 1st ed. (Toronto, ON: Allen Lane, 2017).
2 World Health Organization, *Closing the Gap in a Generation: Health Equity
   through Action on the Social Determinants of Health* (Geneva, Switzerland:
   WHO Press, 2008), accessed March 17, 2017, http://www.who.int/social_
   determinants/thecommission/finalreport/en/.
3 Andre Raynauld and Jean-Pierre Vidal, "Smokers' Burden on Society:
   Myth and Reality in Canada," *Canadian Public Policy* 18, no. 3 (1992):
   18, accessed March 17, 2017, http://www.jstor.org/stable/3551814.
4 Jessica Reid, David Hammond, Vicki L. Rynard, and Robin Burkhalter,
   Tobacco Use in Canada: Patterns and Trends, 2015 ed. (Waterloo, ON:
   Propel Centre for Population Health Impact, University of Waterloo,
   2015), accessed March 17, 2017, https://uwaterloo.ca/tobacco-use
   -canada/tobacco-use-canada-patterns-and-trends
5 Robert Schwartz, Shawn O'Connor, Nadia Minian, Tracey Borland, Alexey
   Babayan, Roberta Ferrence, Joanna Cohen, and Jolene Dubray, *Evidence to
   Inform Smoking Cessation Policymaking in Ontario: A Special Report by the
   Ontario Tobacco Research Unit* (Toronto, ON: Ontario Tobacco Research
   Unit, 2010), accessed March 17, 2017, http://otru.org/wp-content

/uploads/2012/06/special_CAP_august2010.pdf; Canadian Public Health Association, *The Winnable Battle: Ending Tobacco Use in Canada* (Ottawa, ON: Canadian Public Health Association, 2011), accessed March 17, 2017, http://www.cpha.ca/uploads/positions/position-paper-tobacco_e.pdf.

6 Canadian Medical Association, *Health Quality and the Social Determinants of Health* (Ottawa, ON: Canadian Medical Association, 2016), accessed March 17, 2017, https://www.cma.ca/En/Pages/health-equity.aspx; Ryan Meili, *Canada's Doctors Call for Action on Healthy Equity* (Winnipeg, MB: Evidence Network, 2013) [May 2016], accessed March 17, 2017, http://evidencenetwork.ca/archives/13495; Denise Kouri, *Learning from Others: Health Equity Strategies and Initiatives from Canadian Regional Health Authorities* (Toronto, ON: Wellesley Institute, 2013), accessed March 17, 2017, http://www.wellesleyinstitute.com/wp-content/uploads/2013/05/Learning-From-Others.pdf.

7 Health Council of Canada, *Where You Live Matters*.

8 Karen Davis, Kristof Stremikis, David Squires, and Cathy Schoen, *Mirror, Mirror on the Wall: How the Performance of the US Health Care System Compares Internationally* (Washington, DC: Commonwealth Fund, 2014), accessed March 16, 2017, http://www.commonwealthfund.org/~/media/files/publications/fund-report/2014/jun/1755_davis_mirror_mirror_2014.pdf.

9 Elizabeth Parkin, *NHS Maximum Waiting Times Standards and Patient Choice Policies: Briefing Paper Number 07171* (London, England: House of Commons Library, 2016), accessed March 17, 2017, http://researchbriefings.files.parliament.uk/documents/CBP-7171/CBP-7171.pdf.

10 Canadian Institute for Health Information, *Benchmarks for Treatment and Wait Time Trending across Canada* (Ottawa, ON: CIHI, 2016), accessed March 17, 2017, http://waittimes.cihi.ca/; Canadian Institute for Health Information, *Wait Times for Priority Procedures in Canada, 2016* (Ottawa, ON: CIHI, 2016), accessed March 17, 2017, https://secure.cihi.ca/estore/productFamily.htm?pf=PFC3108&lang=en&media=0; Canadian Institute for Health Information, *Access and Wait Times* (Ottawa, ON: CIHI, 2016), accessed March 17, 2017, https://www.cihi.ca/en/health-system-performance/access-and-wait-times.

11 Wait Time Alliance, *Position Paper on the Occasion of the 10th Anniversary of the 2004 10-Year Plan to Strengthen Health Care in Canada: Timely Access to Care for All Canadians: The Role of the Federal Government* (Ottawa, ON: The Alliance, 2014), accessed March 17, 2017, http://www.waittimealliance.ca/wp-content/uploads/2014/09/WTA-Fall-Event-2014-Position-Paper-English-FINAL.pdf; Wait Time Alliance, *Eliminating Code Gridlock in Canada's Health Care System. 2015 Wait Time Alliance*

Report Card (Ottawa, ON: Wait Time Alliance, 2015), accessed March 17, 2017, http://www.waittimealliance.ca/wta-reports/2015-wta-report-card/.

12 Organisation for Economic Co-operation and Development, *Wait Times* (Paris, France: OECD, 2016), accessed March 17, 2017, http://www.oecd.org/els/health-systems/waiting-times.htm.

13 Bacchus Barua, *Waiting Your Turn: Wait Times for Health Care in Canada, 2015 Report* (Toronto, ON: The Fraser Institute, 2015), accessed March 17, 2017, https://www.fraserinstitute.org/studies/waiting-your-turn-wait-times-for-health-care-in-canada-2015-report.

14 John Blake, Daniel Bolland, Ian Dawe, Brenda Gamble, Gunita Mitera, Natalie (Wajs) Rashkovan, Somayeh Sadat, Kenneth Van Wyk, and Raisa Deber, "What to Do with the Queue? Reducing Wait Times for Cancer Care," in *Case Studies in Canadian Health Policy and Management*, 2nd ed., ed. Raisa B. Deber and Catherine L. Mah, (Toronto, ON: University of Toronto Press, 2014), 312–28.

15 Saskatchewan Surgical Initiative, *Pooled Referrals: Guide for Referring Health Providers* (Regina, SK: Government of Saskatchewan, 2016), accessed March 17, 2017, http://www.sasksurgery.ca/provider/pooledreferrals.html.

16 The Centre for Healthcare Engineering at the University of Toronto has undertaken a number of such projects. *About Us* (Toronto, ON: University of Toronto, Faculty of Applied Science & Engineering, 2017), accessed March 17, 2017, http://che.utoronto.ca/us/.

17 Choosing Wisely Canada, *Home Page* (Toronto, ON: Choose Wisely, 2016), accessed March 17, 2017, http://www.choosingwiselycanada.org/.

18 G. Ross Baker, "Governance, Policy and System-Level Efforts to Support Safer Healthcare," *Healthcare Quarterly* 17, Special Issue (2014): 21–6, http://www.longwoods.com/content/23955.

19 Terrence Sullivan and Adalsteinn Brown, "Inching towards Accountability for Quality: Early Days for the Excellent Care for All Act," *Healthcare Management Forum* 27, no. 2 (2014): 56–9, accessed March 17, 2017, http://www.sciencedirect.com/science/article/pii/S0840470414000441.

20 Raisa B. Deber, "Thinking about Accountability," *Healthcare Policy* 10, Special (2014): 12–24, accessed March 17, 2017, http://www.longwoods.com/content/23932 (see also the other articles in this special issue of the journal); Approaches to Accountability, *Home Page* (Toronto, ON: Approaches to Accountability Research Team, 2016), accessed March 17, 2017, http://www.approachestoaccountability.ca/.

21 Derick W. Brinkerhoff, "Accountability and Health Systems: Toward Conceptual Clarity and Policy Relevance," *Health Policy and Planning* 19,

no. 6 (2004): 371–9, http://heapol.oxfordjournals.org/cgi/reprint /19/6/371.

22 Linda T. Kohn, Janet M. Corrigan, and Molla S. Donaldson, *To Err Is Human: Building a Safer Health System* (Washington, DC: National Academy Press, 2000).

23 Peter C. Smith, Elias Mossialos, Irene Papanicolas, and Sheila Leatherman, eds., *Performance Measurement for Health System Improvement: Experiences, Challenges and Prospects* (Cambridge, MA: Cambridge University Press, 2009); Robert Schwartz, Alex Price, Raisa B. Deber, Heather Manson, and Fran Scott, "Hopes and Realities of Public Health Accountability Policies," *Healthcare Policy* 10, Special Issue (2014): 79–89, http://www.longwoods.com/content/23916.

24 Robert Schwartz and Raisa Deber, "The Performance Measurement – Management Divide in Public Health," *Health Policy* 120, no. 3 (2016): 273–80; Raisa Deber and Robert Schwartz, "What's Measured Is Not Necessarily What Matters: A Cautionary Story from Public Health," *Healthcare Policy* 12, no. 2 (2016): 52–64, http://www.sciencedirect.com /science/article/pii/S0168851016300033.

25 Health Council of Canada, *Better Health, Better Care, Better Value for All: Refocusing Health Care Reform in Canada* (Toronto, ON: Health Council of Canada, 2013), accessed March 17, 2017, http://www.healthcouncilcanada .ca/content_bh.php?mnu=2&mnu1=48&mnu2=30&mnu3=53.

26 The Health Council of Canada reports remain available online for reference purposes through Carleton University Library, accessed March 17, 2017, http://www.healthcouncilcanada.ca.

8   Treating Health Care: How Can We Make It Better? What Might Make It Worse?

1 Juha Mikkonen and Dennis Raphael, *Social Determinants of Health: The Canadian Facts* (Toronto, ON: York University School of Health Policy and Management, 2010), accessed March 17, 2017, http://www .thecanadianfacts.org/.

2 Leatt, Pink, and Guerriere, "Towards a Canadian Model of Integrated Healthcare."

3 Emma Wallace, Chris Salisbury, Bruce Guthrie, Cliona Lewis, Tom Fahey, and Susan M. Smith, "Clinical Review: Managing Patients with Multimorbidity in Primary Care," *BMJ* 350 (2015), http://www.bmj.com /content/350/bmj.h176.

4 Considerable information about EHRs is available from the Canada Health Infoway site, accessed March 17, 2017. https://www.infoway -inforoute.ca/en/.

5 Raisa Deber and Noralou Roos, "Making Patients Pay Won't Make Our Health System More Affordable," in *Canadian Health Policy in the News: Why Evidence Matters*, ed. Noralou Roos, Sharon Manson Singer, and Kathleen O'Grady (Winnipeg, MA: Evidence Network, 2012), 332–4, http://evidencenetwork.ca/archives/4380.

6 Raisa Deber, Evelyn Forget, and Leslie L. Roos, "Medical Savings Accounts in a Universal System: Wishful Thinking Meets Evidence," *Health Policy* 70, no. 1 (2004): 49–66, accessed March 17, 2017, https://www.ncbi.nlm .nih.gov/pubmed/15312709; Raisa Deber and Kenneth C.K. Lam, *Medical Savings Accounts in Financing Healthcare*, CHSRF Reports on Financing Models: Paper 3 (Ottawa, ON: CHSRF, 2011), accessed March 17, 2017, http://www.cfhi-fcass.ca/sf-docs/default-source/commissioned-research -reports/RAISA3-MedicalSAcc_EN.pdf?sfvrsn=0; Raisa Deber and Kenneth C.K. Lam, *Experience with Medical Savings Accounts in Selected Jurisdictions*, CHSRF Series of Reports on Financing Models: Paper 4 (Ottawa, ON: CHSRF, 2011), accessed March 17, 2017, http://www.cfhi-fcass.ca /sf-docs/default-source/commissioned-research-reports/RAISA4 _Experience_in_MSA_EN.pdf?sfvrsn=0.

7 Raisa Deber, Alina Gildiner, and Pat Baranek, "Why Not Private Health Insurance? 1. Insurance Made Easy," *Canadian Medical Association Journal* 161, no. 5 (1999): 539–44, accessed March 17, 2017, http://www .cmaj.ca/content/161/5/539.full.text; Raisa Deber, Alina Gildiner, and Pat Baranek, "Why Not Private Health Insurance? 2. Actuarial Principles Meet Provider Dreams," *Canadian Medical Association Journal* 161, no. 5 (1999): 545–50, accessed March 17, 2017, https://www.ncbi.nlm.nih.gov /pubmed/10497614; Raisa Deber, Nathalie St. Pierre, Devidas Menon, and John Wade, "The Use and Misuse of Economics," in *Do We Care? Renewing Canada's Commitment to Health*, ed. Margaret A. Somerville (Montreal, QC: McGill-Queen's University Press, 1999), 53–68; Deber, "Delivering Health Care Services," in *The Fiscal Sustainability of Health Care in Canada*.

8 Standing Senate Committee on Social Affairs Science and Technology, *The Health of Canadians – The Federal Role. Volume Six: Recommendations for Reform*.

9 Commission on the Future of Health Care in Canada, *Building on Values: The Future of Health Care in Canada*.

10 Raisa Deber, Lutchmie Narine, Pat Baranek, Natasha Sharpe, Katya Masnyk Duvalko, Randi Zlotnik-Shaul, Peter Coyte, George Pink, and Paul Williams, "The Public-Private Mix in Health Care," in *Canada Health Action: Building on the Legacy*, ed. National Forum on Health (Sainte-Foy, QC: Éditions MultiMondes, 1998), 423–545.
11 Morgan, Gagnon, Mintzes, and Lexchin, "A Better Prescription."
12 Andrea Gabrielli, Nicolas T. Layon, Holly L. Bones, and Joseph Layon, "The Tragedy of the Commons – Drug Shortages and Our Patients' Health," *American Journal of Medicine* 129, no. 12 (2016): 1237–8.
13 Steven Morgan, Jamie Daw, and Paige Thomson, "International Best Practices for Negotiating 'Reimbursement Contracts' with Price Rebates from Pharmaceutical Companies," *Health Affairs* 32, no. 4 (2013): 771–7, https://www.ncbi.nlm.nih.gov/pubmed/23569058.
14 The Council of the Federation of Canada's Premiers, *The Pan-Canadian Pharmaceutical Alliance* (Ottawa, ON: Council of the Federation Secretariat, 2016), accessed March 17, 2017, http://www.pmprovinces territoires.ca/en/initiatives/358-pan-canadian-pharmaceutical-alliance; Government of Canada, *News Release – Government of Canada Partners with Provinces and Territories to Lower Cost of Pharmaceuticals* (Ottawa, ON: Health Canada, 2015), accessed March 17, 2017, http://news.gc.ca/web/article-en.do?nid=1028339.
15 Steven G. Morgan, Michael R. Law, Jamie R. Daw, Liza Abraham, and Danielle Martin. "Estimated Cost of Universal Public Coverage of Prescription Drugs in Canada," *Canadian Medical Association Journal* 187, no. 7 (2015), Epub March 16, 2015, http://www.cmaj.ca/content/early/2015/03/16/cmaj.141564.
16 Williams, Lum, Morton-Chang, Kuluski, Peckham, Warrick, and Ying, *Integrating Long-Term Care into a Community-Based Continuum.*
17 Steffie Woolhandler, Terry Campbell, and David U. Himmelstein, "Costs of Health Care Administration in the United States and Canada," *New England Journal of Medicine* 349, no. 8 (2003): 768–75.
18 David U. Himmelstein, Miraya Jun, Reinhard Busse, Karine Chevreul, Alexander Geissler, Patrick Jeurissen, Sarah Thomson, Marie-Amelie Vinet, and Steffie Woolhandler, "A Comparison of Hospital Administrative Costs in Eight Nations: US Costs Exceed All Others by Far," *Health Affairs* 33, no. 9 (2014): 1586–94, http://content.healthaffairs.org/content/33/9/1586.abstract.

Index